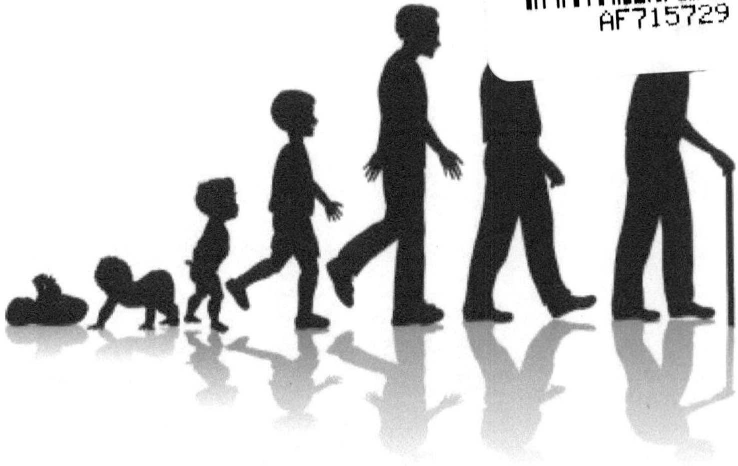

CARE GIVING: REAL LIFE ANSWERS

By

Sydney A. Clary

Paperback ISBN: 9798224546664

eBook Version: 9798224821464

Author: Sydney A. Clary

Book Cover Design: Jolene MacFadden

Table of Contents

AUTHOR'S NOTE

This book is a result of over forty years of caring for others, either in their homes or mine. All of the people involved were relatives and children. Each was unique in his or her needs. When someone, anyone, starts a job with no training and next to nothing out there for resource information, you either learn quickly or you run screaming from the room. I'm not a runner but, more importantly, I could not desert those around me who needed help. Equally, I am not a martyr. I wanted a life too. I had a husband, and, within three years, I had children. I didn't want to give up time with them to take care of someone else no matter how much I cared. I had to find a way to do it all and not end up needing a caregiver myself.

Everything written here is a result, a solution that has stood the test of time and experience in my world. Your world is different. Some of the things exactly as they are presented may help you, some may simply give you an idea that you hadn't considered but may work better in your situation.

I am no expert, and I won't pretend to be one. Yet hardly a week goes by, without a friend or a friend of a friend asking me 'what do I do here'. After years of nagging of friends and my family when they were still with me, I created this book. I have given it to other care givers to read before it was printed. A book like this is no good to anyone if it doesn't actually work. I was stunned at the reaction. There were tears, a number of 'I wish I had thought of that', 'I wish I had known that' from those who had already been through their caregiving years. From those who hadn't started there was a single, consistent response, 'When is the book coming out and how do I get a copy?'

So, with those responses in mind I stepped out of my comfort zone of fiction writing and stepped Care Giving: Real Life Answers. This is not a textbook or reference manual format. This is a book about people, real people, like you and like me. Care giving, in my opinion, isn't about the chores and the doctor appointments and the living arrangements as much as it is about the lives of the care giver and the person or persons who need help. Because of this, there are examples sprinkled throughout the book. Most are my relatives. Every one of them of so different and approached aging with all those differences creating bridges and obstacles that made care giving a course in mental, emotional and physical gymnastics. That aspect is clear in these pages.

I hope this book helps you in whatever stage of care giving you are. For most of us, running screaming from the room as we face this time of life isn't an option. You can have a life, personal, professional and social. It takes planning, ingenuity and creativity. If you have a bit of humor that can really help too. You can do this successfully and still have a life. It isn't easy. It is blood, sweat and tears but it is doable. In my case, I found there was laughter and loving and a special closeness I wouldn't have had any other way.

CHAPTER ONE

WHAT IS CAREGIVING?

This seems a simple enough question with a simple answer. There are two basic age groups of care giving, children and adults. This book is focused mainly on the adult care giving situation. I was the mother of a learning-disabled child during the years when I was caring for adults. I found that many of the strategies I developed worked with her in similar situations. Where those apply in this book, I will comment. I have no experience with a child with severe problems, mental, physical or emotional. However, it is possible that some of the situations and solutions will spawn ideas for you if that is the situation you are facing.

When one is talking about being a care giver for children, we have a fairly good idea of what that entails. Mention care giving for a mother, father or grandparent in a roomful of people and everyone will give a different answer and most of those will be shaded with the burden each person feels as he or she considers the active aspect of doing it daily or with the fear of having to be a care giver in the future.

Most of us fear dying. Most of us don't want to see those who matter to us dying.

And that is what the word care giving often invokes in us. Think about it.

When about-to-be parents consider the road stretched before them with care giving there is a sense of anticipation and wonder, excitement and, yes, a little fear. But the fear here has a more positive ring.

As I struggle to write about this aspect, really the first step of care giving for an aging relative or special friend, I can thank a friend of mine who insisted this should be one of the first things to address in this book. This woman and I raised our children together. She has watched me deal with my family and my husband's family. She has called repeatedly with questions from her friends about their struggles.

Dying almost always rears its inevitable head. I took a class on dying once. The professor, a man who looked to be in his sixties and was really in his late eighties, said something that I thought was very profound.

"We start dying from our first breath."

Anyone who was intending to snooze through that class woke up with a jerk. Comments ranged from the joke of two things are guaranteed in life, death and taxes, to how can you say that?

He was right. We are all dying, today, tomorrow, next week, fifty years from now. None of us know when death may strike or some illness or accident that will incapacitate us. More importantly, there is no way to escape departing this world. Death is as much a part of living as birth is. Yet, in this country for the most part, we shun the thought of death, fight to stay young, look young and feel young. Aging is that dreaded condition of misery and helplessness that scares us to death. We nip and tuck, diet and exercise, shove pills of all kinds down our throats in an effort to hold the inevitable at bay. And when we look at our loved ones facing this time, we carry this fear, this anger, this frustration into the care giving process whether we know it or not.

We are not one of the world's cultures that actually respect and reveres aging and age. Believe it or not, there are people who see the richness of this time not the decay. I am not trying to tell anyone how to face this time, but I am hoping you will begin to understand your own feelings and your loved ones as well. Both sides are living with this in the back of the mind and in the heart. Your loved one feels the burden he or she is placing on you. You feel the burden too. Neither of you want this situation that life has thrust on you.

But is this the only way to approach care giving? I don't think so. This long-ago class started me thinking in new ways. Okay, death was the end but what about all the time before that moment? How did I want to live it? How could I help my loved ones to live it?

I was already taking care of my husband's family with his help. Weekly, we were making the trip, thirty odd miles one way, two babies with us, to clean, shop and do yard work. In those years, because medical insurance was spotty at best and our children had medical conditions that cost a great deal in special foods and ER trips, my husband even worked a second job. We had no spare time, but we loved his father and mother.

Does this, at least in part, sound familiar?

I had been feeling the crush of exhaustion, the worry about my husband's heavy schedule, my children's health and watching his family fade, knowing that soon Papa and Mama Clary would not be with us and that, one day I would be watching my family walk the same path. As I listened to the professor discuss death, I found life was more important. I found that I could see each day as a gift, one more sunrise of having those we loved near. Maybe I was tired, but I had time to chat while I washed dishes. I had time to laugh with my mother-in-law while my children learned to walk to the couch where Mama Clary lay because her heart was slowly giving out.

I had time to pick the vegetables and fruits Papa Clary could grow with all ten of his green thumbs. The two of us together would blanch and freeze the abundance, halving it for his freezer and mine. I learned from him even as I was doing much of the work he could no longer do. When I needed bookshelves, my father-in-law was a master carpenter, he came tools in hand and built them for me. The first set was done in is sixties, the second in his seventies and the third and final in his eighties. All through those twenty years, my husband and helped him but he helped us too. If I and my husband hadn't taken on the task of care giving, we would have missed all those moments.

Because of the professor, I could begin to see the gift not the burden most days. I'm no saint so every day wasn't that glowing, but most were. It was amazing to realize, some months later, that I no longer felt as tired even though I was slowly taking on more work. I made another discovery; **attitude can make a huge difference**.

And this brings me to one of my few pet peeves, *parenting the parent*. This approach really should be revisited. When someone parents a child, that child has always been dependent on that person, he has never known independence. He looks to his parent automatically, through imprinting and training, to find his safety, his comfort and his security. An adult, one who has cared for you, wiped your nose, held your hand, loaned you money, listened to your troubles, is exactly the opposite, in my opinion.

The chances of your mother or father happily settling in to being organized, prodded ever so gently or even not so gently, or worse, told what to do by you when his or her body is failing but the mind is still sharp, aren't too great. Neither likes being dependent, and each likes it even less when each is feeling death creeping closer. He or she is losing even the illusion of control over his or her own body. Doctors' appointments, medications around the clock and you standing in the background parenting are **NOT** a good prescription for a happy life for any of you.

An example right here is a bit funny in hindsight, but it certainly was traumatic in the moment. Papa Clary had fruit trees in his tiny back yard. The orange tree was laden with the best oranges. He called my husband and asked him to harvest the fruit. It was mid-week and David was working overtime so he told his father he would be there first thing on Saturday as usual and he would get the fruit in before he did anything else.

My father-in-law decided not to wait. Late afternoon, he put a ladder up in the center of the tree to pick the fruit. He fell through the tree.

Thankfully it was only about twelve feet tall, and the branches broke his fall, but they also ripped his ears off his cute little bald head. I received the call from the emergency room. David had just arrived home from work and dropped into bed for a quick nap. He had just worked about twelve hours. I woke him and he raced for the hospital while I stayed with the children.

The rest of this tale. according to both men, went like this.

David: "You had no business getting on a ladder at your age. I told you I would pick the damn oranges."

Papa Clary: "Son, I knew you were working. I didn't like bothering you and the fruit was ripening."

David: "You could have killed yourself. If you don't promise me that you'll stay out of the tree, I'll cut the damn thing down."

Papa Clary: "It's my house and my tree. If I want to climb it, I will."

My husband rarely cursed but he did that night. My father-in-law rarely confronted anyone, but he went toe to toe with his son over those oranges. Neither was given to sulking, but they gave new meaning to the word for the next week. Eventually, they made peace. David did the harvesting, or I did. And Papa Clary's ears grew back thanks to a really good surgeon.

The moral of this story is: don't expect your relative to listen like a child does most of the time. The next time, the ears may not grow back.

Quality of life is critical for the person for whom you are caring currently or going to be. It is also critical, for you especially, if you have a full house, a career and a social life. When either side of this partnership, the person needing care or the one giving it, has to give something up, the other side is going to know it too. Resentments are born here on both sides. Guilt is not an idea any longer, it is a fact. Most of the time, it can seem, from both sides, that one side is trying to **control the other**. Fighting, verbally or silently, to be the one calling the shots can become an issue**. It is not about parenting when you are dealing with an adult who has been independent**. It is about working together to find solutions that work for both of you.

Finally, thankfully, there are more resources available for those of us who are care giving. I will do my best to reference any I have used. Every state is different, unfortunately. However, the internet and some well spent time make reaching out easier than it has ever been to date.

CHAPTER TWO

SETTING UP A RELATIONSHIP

The first time I started care giving, the process didn't even have a name. My husband and I just got a simple phone call: 'Son, I'm having a little trouble with the kitchen sink. Could you look at it for me?'

Papa Clary was a very independent man and very handy with tools, but he was already seventy-four when we married. Getting down on the floor and scrunched inside the kitchen cabinet under the sink to get to the piping to the faucet just wasn't possible anymore. He could have called a plumber, but he knew we were coming to our weekly supper anyway. David didn't mind dealing with it and would have been upset if his dad had called a plumber when he could fix the problem easily enough.

This one call opened the door for helping out. We were happy to do it. We both loved his parents and they asked very little and were always patient, not counting the orange tree episode, until we could get there. But the list kept growing. Now we had children, first one then, twenty-three months later, another. Those children had severe medical issues. David had to work two jobs just to make ends meet. Time was a commodity we didn't have. By now, we were deep in care giving. His mother's heart was giving out. His father was eighty and the list was growing.

This is how it begins for so many of us. That one call for help. My husband and I didn't know enough, didn't even realize what we were doing and if there was even a casually accepted name for the situation in which we found ourselves we didn't know it. On the job training was the order of the day. We fumbled our way through, worrying about small stuff, missing some things like the orange tree and wearing ourselves out. A great deal of the stress and strain could have been mitigated if we had simply addressed the situation with his parents. They loved us. They needed us and they weren't unreasonable.

Eventually, David and I talked to them. That first dialogue had us both scared, me more than my husband. He was the much more laid back of the two of us. We set up a plan of action that suited the four of us and implemented it. The impossible, unwieldy, time consuming tasks we had been handling became much less time consuming and much more manageable. We still had to make two trips a week, seventy miles each, but we didn't end up with lists we just couldn't complete. This first sit down taught me a valuable lesson that I use to this day with any problem that involves someone else.

MAKE THE FIRST CONFERENCE INFORMAL AND PLEASUREABLE In other words, don't make a "I have to talk to you" announcement. Everyone, you included braces for trouble in this kind of setting. This first chat sets the tone. I, for one, find it easier to work with someone when we both want to **be heading in the same direction.** You want to help, or you wouldn't have accepted that first indication or call that said I need help from someone I care about. The person, mother, father or relative who asks, cares about you, trusts you enough that he or she is reaching out.

Example: Our first ever talk happened over dinner. "What can we do to really help ya'll? (Did I mention, we're as southern as we can stare?) We feel like we're leaving things out that you need just because we aren't planning very well. What can we do to make it easier for all of us, especially since when we come, we want to have time to visit too?" Keep in mind the calls on your own time, job, partner, children, etc.

DIALOGUE In the brief account above, you'll see we were inviting dialogue. I can't take credit for realizing or even planning it at the time. We didn't. It was only later, when I heard adult children like us stepping in to help their parents that most had used what I call the "I'll take care of it or you need to do this" approach with no input from the person needing help.

Your loved one needs help from **someone who matters to them, not a commander of the troops**. Explain the situation as you see it. Explain what you think you can do to help and, most importantly, when. This sounds too simple to be important. I believe this is critical. You can't help effectively if you don't understand what is needed. Chances are what you think you see as a problem may not be it at all.

ASK QUESTIONS Remember this is a dialogue. Get input. It's his/her needs that you are trying to meet. This part is going to occur more than once as your loved one ages. Changes in health are usually the motivating factors but finances can play a part as well. It is important to be aware as the changes happen in your loved one's life so that you can respond to the new situation. Do your best to keep the dialogue open between you. Talk as honestly as possible with your loved one. In an ideal world, complete honesty would be the rule but in these sensitive family dynamics that is not always the case. In other words, think before you speak and choose your words with care. This is a difficult time. Be kind to yourself and your loved one.

LISTEN If you don't understand what you are hearing say so. This is a dialogue not a monologue. I don't think there was a single person in my care who wasn't strong willed and stubborn. This one simple thing, listening, made dealing with each of them easier.

IF WHAT HE OR SHE WANTS DOESN'T WORK FOR YOU EXPLAIN WHY. Again, dialogue is the key. The person you are caring for cares about you whether he or she expresses it or not. It takes a great deal for an independent person to knowingly put himself in another person's hands. He or she wants this to work but more than that, **he or she needs it to work.**

FIND A COMPROMISE This part may take some work especially because most of us want the sweetest part of the deal. Whenever I got to this point, I thought fifty-fifty and made sure I knew, and he/she knew what each of us was getting and giving up.

Example: My parents and I shared the same clothes washer and dryer. I certainly didn't wash clothes every day and neither did they. I discussed this issue with them, and we selected a couple of days for each of us. My mother was not the most accommodating woman in the universe so, shortly after, we both ended up at the machine not only on the same day but the same hour.

I found her stuffing clothes in the washer on my day. It wasn't the first time, usually she managed to have started the load before I discovered her scheduling change. Now, looking at the clothes packed in the washer was the final straw moment.

I said, "Okay, I'll do mine tomorrow from now on."

Surprised, she stopped filling the tub long enough to look at me. "But that is the day you take me shopping."

Sometimes silence is better than words. She got the point. She unloaded the washer and decided to stick to the routine we had decided on together. Shopping trumped laundry.

AVOID ARGUING There are so many ways to get a point across without going to war. For me, anger is the hardest emotion to deal with when care giving. It seems like no one can hear anything through this one emotion. Reason is ten times harder to achieve and that's on a good day. Also, few if any of us, guard our words when we're angry. Once the person you are caring for has said ugly things to you, you aren't going to feel like accommodating him/her or, if you do, you are resenting everything you do. **Try to get ahead of situations that can escalate into fights**. You won't win and neither will he/she. Talk about the problem. Open the discussion. No matter what it is, remember this person matters to you or you wouldn't have taken this person into your life this way.

TAKE THE WORK OUT OF CARE GIVING This one is going to require a bit of ingenuity and planning. Again, working with the one for whom you are caring is the key. **Example:** My father had a standing appointment for having his blood drawn once a month. The order was for fasting lab work. He had diabetes and was taking blood thinners, so it was important that he didn't miss this appointment and, as a diabetic it was important, that his meal schedule be consistent. Adding the two together, when the lab opened at 7:30 am was the best time to take him. I certainly didn't want to hop out of bed, shove myself into clothes and so forth then jump in the car after having loaded him and drive twenty miles to the lab. However, we both liked breakfast and shopping early at the supermarket. So instead of being annoyed about the 7:30 am appointment, we made an outing out of it. We handled the blood draw then had a leisurely breakfast I didn't have to cook after which we shopped for groceries when the store wasn't crowded. Not all problems are this easy to solve but most do have solutions if you just take a few moments to stop and think. You are busy. A few minutes of thought often saves hours in work.

TAKE CARE OF THE CARE GIVER That's you! We who are care givers are not machines or super powered men and women. WE GET TIRED, FED UP AND DEFEATED. Care giving is demanding on every level. I personally think the emotional and mental strain far exceeds the physical one.

Take breaks. Please, don't give me the argument, I can't. Yes, you can. Respite care is possible, through churches, through friends, through relatives or through home health organizations. Some have a cost, and some do not. Taking breaks takes planning and preparation but it is necessary. If you end up sick or in the hospital yourself, someone is going to have to step in anyway and you'll get a break but you sure won't enjoy it or reap the benefit of recharging.

Vent when necessary. Caregiving creates all kinds of conflicts even in the best of us. Having someone you trust, someone who can listen is special in any kind of relationship but, in this area, I found it critical. I was lucky enough to have two women, one who had been a care giver before me and one who had not. In both cases, I could trust them to not only listen to my tale of woe but to respond with ideas or simple sympathy. And no, I was not always right in the way that I handled things. They were the kind of friends who could point me in the right direction, and I trusted them enough to consider each suggestion, either using it as given or tweaking it to fit the situation.

Support groups exist in some areas to answer this need. Organizations such as Hospice often offer counselling services. Even if you are someone who would ordinarily not choose this way, I'm that kind of personality, I would suggest you at least consider the idea and maybe check out the possibilities. The benefit to both you and your loved one may far exceed what you could imagine.

BE AWARE OF YOUR RESOURCES You do have them, and I will do my best in later chapters to give you starting points on those that I know as well.

HAVE COPIES OF ALL IMPORTANT PAPERWORK Even if this is your first phone call for help or if you know that call is in the future, you should have the paperwork in hand for handling your loved one's affairs if necessary. Illness or accident can happen at any time with no warning. If you are going to be the one doing the care giving you will legally need documents that clearly outline your rights and responsibilities. Your relative may not even have these documents. Find out. A crisis is not the time to be digging in drawers looking for a power of attorney or a DNR.

I know setting up a relationship sounds complicated but in reality, most of this can be initially accomplished in an hour or so of frank discussion with two willing parties. More discussions will probably occur along the way but having set up the first successful dialogue, communication should be easier. Again, keep in mind the personalities of those with whom you are talking. Don't forget yourself. Honesty and kindness added to the connection between you and those who need you is more valuable than you realize

CHAPTER THREE

CARE FACILITY OR HOME?

Where you are doing the care giving affects everything you do. If you work, most do, travel time is lost time in many ways. It isn't shortening your list or the list of those for whom you are caring. Those minutes, hours spent getting to your loved one give the care giver plenty of time to second guess actions or words, both about what he/she has taken on but what he/she has let go to take on this time consuming task. Few, if any of us, realize how this worry time can affect what we are doing. I didn't at first. It took months before I yanked myself up short and realized I often arrived either at my in-laws in a fever of energy to get things done so I could get home. Or got home so tired and defeated by the huge task of virtually running two households I wanted to just pull the covers over my head and pretend I didn't know anyone.

Once I realized I was making a hard job even more difficult, I used the thirty-mile trip for me. My husband and I loved music. It's relaxing but we definitely didn't have time to sit and listen to any with our schedule. However, the car had a tape deck back in the day. We picked out tapes we liked and suspended conversation on those trips back and forth. I was amazed at what the simple solution did for both of us.

The point here is that care giving is very demanding and you, as the care giver, are under a lot of stress in areas you won't necessarily see immediately. When you do, don't ignore those moments. Find a way that works for you and deal with them. Stress is cumulative and debilitating.

Now, let's talk about the location aspect of care giving. There are three basic sites: in the home of the person or persons who need you, your home or a facility of some sort. Bringing your loved into your home will have Chapter Four all to itself. I will address the relative's home and care facility here.

Facilities come in a range of types and quality of care depending on the state. There are rules governing all of them. None of the care facilities are meant to take the place of family. They are meant to assist the family in taking care of those who can no longer take care of themselves. There are two basic types with variations on those as well.

Nursing home—In some places this is called extended care. This is a 24/7 nursing care situation. A doctor or doctors see the patients on a regular basis. Meals, baths and various skilled medical services are provided such as physical therapy, occupational therapy, respiratory support, etc. Most offer support for family members and regular conferences to discuss needs and goals. There are costs involved with this care. Depending on the insurance of your loved one, Medicare and/or a supplement, the costs can be prohibitive. Check with the insurances involved before you begin your research.

Assisted Living There are so many kinds of this particular care that to name them all would be lengthy. The facility can be as simple as a basic motel design with everyone in a private room to more elaborate set ups with individual small homes or villas. Some have permanent nursing staff, some don't. Most offer meals, laundry service, hair care, banking, shopping and excursions to town or cultural events, etc. The cost to the individual is greater here and the insurance, unless specialized just for this, doesn't cover much if anything. Extra services such as hair care and laundry are additional costs.

Fortunately, with the internet, there is so much research available on so many sites, that when the need arises you can make an informed choice about what is right for you and your loved one. However, research on the net or just talking with experts or those in the field is not enough. Check out the facility yourself. A pamphlet is not enough. Word of mouth is not enough. Quality varies and your loved one is a person with likes and dislikes. Below are tips on what to look for and most of all the questions to ask.

The lobby area, if there is one, is staged to give the best appearance to the visitor. Ask to see a room or villa. I have actually been in some facilities that won't allow this. For me, that is a red flag. I want to know if the room is a cubby hole or a room with space to move. Is there television? A phone? A window? What is the view like?

Your loved one is going to be living here for an indeterminate time. Essentially this is going to be their home. Is there clothes storage? A place for pictures? A chair for visitors? Some places I have seen have bare minimum in furniture but allow the family to bring in a few things. If you don't see the things that would be important to your loved one, ask if you can supply them.

Pay attention to the smell. If it smells like an unclean bathroom it probably is no matter how attractive the décor. If it reeks of pine cleaner there is a reason. Staph infections are a very real concern in modern care facilities. Cleanliness decreases the risk.

Check the bathroom area Is there an emergency cord in easy reach? Are there grab bars in the shower. Do the fixtures look clean and in good repair? Is the linen, towels, etc. clean, unfrayed and stain free? Is the area big enough in which to move? Is it in the room or down the hall?

Do those on staff address the residents by name? Does the resident respond with pleasure and a smile? If asked a question, does your guide stop to answer or just brush the resident off?

Example: When my father-in-law started having mini strokes, the doctor wanted him in a care facility. I had the task of checking out the places. One of them, highly recommended, looked to be the best on paper. I hated it. I was there thirty minutes and I didn't see one resident smiling or talking to the care givers. I didn't see one member of the staff stop and address a resident by name and the guide I had had four opportunities to answer questions and she brushed every one off and even explained that you had to be firm with old people.

I have been in other facilities where the guides knew every resident and made a point of stopping and asking questions about a book they were reading, a class they were taking. The guide waited for an answer and even asked another question. Yes, this could have been just good PR but I doubt it simply because how can one person know who was going to be coming into the lobby at any given moment and just what they might be reading or doing?

Part of the job of this kind of care facility is to give your loved one a version of the lifestyle that he/she can no longer have alone. Good ones do a really great job with this. Bad ones make aging hell. Since you signed the papers, you get to carry some if not all of the responsibility of having placed someone you care about in the care of others who do not care. Do your research.

If possible, have a meal. lunch or breakfast is a good test. Nutrition is critical but if the food doesn't taste good, isn't plated to look good, no one feels like eating well. Are snacks available and what are they generally? What about holiday meals? Can you take your relative out to lunch? Can they have guests in? Can you provide food?

Additional Services Hair care, shaves, laundry, shopping and entertainment excursions. Get a list with costs. In nursing home settings, most of these will be included or not appropriate for your loved one's state of health. Check anyway. No one, aged or not, wants to stare at the same walls all day with nothing to do. Any services not provided on site will be your responsibility. Often, the more the person ages, the more difficult and time consuming it will become to take outside trips. Figure those possibilities into the cost of the facility's care.

Check the grounds. Are there areas for walking? A pool? Gardens? If you have a relative who loves being outside, don't ignore that need if at all possible. Look for some place with an outdoor area that is accessible to the residents.

Example: The last time my husband was in a care facility, one surrounded by beautiful green grass and bird feeders at every window, I watched a very pretty lady wheel her chair every morning to this glass door at the end of the hall. She would sit there for hours just looking out. This facility didn't have any walks outside.

It didn't matter in my husband's case as he was bed ridden but she was not. She had tears in her eyes when she told me about her flowers and her gardens. She missed them so much and she couldn't go outside anymore because no one had time to wheel her down the single sidewalk that flanked the building on two sides. She loved when her family visited. They took her out in the parking lot and on that one sidewalk.

This facility was not a good match for her. Less than three blocks away there was a care facility that had walks and a moss draped tree shaded landscape. This facility allowed the residents outside. In fact, it even organized small outdoor events a couple of times a year. Since I had checked both out, I knew the cost was almost the same. There could have been reasons that the family responsible for this lady had not chosen the other place or somewhere better suited for their relative. Obviously, I didn't have the whole story. However, equally possible somehow, someone either didn't know or hadn't asked what this lady needed. As a care giver you won't get everything right but something this basic should not have happened.

Does the facility offer outside trips? Many do. Things from shopping to cultural events can be on the list. If you have a relative that likes dining out see if that can be arranged if it isn't on the regular schedule. Most things like this can be with advanced planning.

Remember this is your loved one's new home. You want him or her to be happy and to enjoy his or her new life as much as possible.

Does the facility offer the basics, such as a banking representative on site, a pharmacy, a place to purchase items like Kleenex, toothpaste, etc.? Many have small stores for the residents' convenience. The prices are a little higher, but this gives your loved one some independence and saves you some time running errands.

Can your loved one take day trips or even overnight trips? Many facilities do offer this, and it can be very rewarding for everyone. Birthdays, holidays, family reunions are all possible reasons or even just because you miss them.

Finally, pay attention to what you see and hear when you visit your loved one. Most of all listen to what he/she says. If your loved one is happy you will know it. If not, find out why. Talk to the staff to see if there is a resolution. Aging should not be a prison with you holding the key. There is a reason why your loved one is here but there is no reason his or her stay can't be as pleasant as possible.

The next site is your loved one's home. He/she wants to stay there. You live somewhere else. If you are caring for a couple or a single, you are still going to worry about all the what ifs.

Consider discussing with your loved one an alert device. There are many companies offering these now. The prices vary and the range of use as well. These devices are worn pendant style or on the wrist. Although, neither is a fashion statement, having one on means that should your relative fall in the shower, in the bedroom etc., all that is needed is to press a button to let someone know the problem. The company then dials 911 to dispatch emergency help and, since they have your loved one's medical history and medications, they can transfer any data necessary for optimum care. Companies offer 24/7 monitoring, and many have alarms, fire and burglary, that can be added to the home.

Contracts can be involved so research each company carefully. It only takes one fall and the resulting broken bones to move from being independent to very dependent, sometimes permanently dependent. This one statement is often the tide turning argument if your loved one refuses to consider the device.

Assess your loved one's home with a new eye. What works for a person in his thirties or forties often doesn't in the seventies and eighties. There are experts who can do this for you if you don't have the time or feel you aren't skilled enough. If you want to do the assessment yourself, here are some tips.

Check for smoke alarms, carbon monoxide alarms and a security system if the area is not as safe as you would like. There are a number of versions of these that can either hook into existing electrical systems, I would suggest a professional here, or are battery operated and attached to ceilings or walls. The direct hook ups also have batteries. This will be one more thing on your list to check yearly and replace batteries.

Check accessibility. If your loved one is using any kind of mobility aid, walker, wheelchair, cane, he/she will find getting around in the average house difficult. Most interior doors are not 36 inches wide and it is possible, depending on the age of the home, that the exterior door isn't either. This is the suggested width and, especially in the case of a wheelchair, the necessary width for mobility. If your relative is not in a chair, he/she can certainly try to maneuver through the narrow doorway but in doing so the very device that could aid them then becomes an issue. Changing a door opening size is a job for a professional.

Clutter. Mom or Dad may love their clutter, but it also means clear paths from one room or area to the next are hard to find. You don't have to go crazy here, but you could suggest display cabinets or areas rather than the shotgun effect. Depending on your schedule and finances and the size of the task you may want to consider a professional to take on this aspect. However, if this is the best choice for you as the care giver, a discussion that involves an agreement to the changes you want to make for your relative will make the situation easier on everyone.

Also, make a detailed list for the company or yourself on the areas to address. It is very easy in this kind of process to clear one area and make another more difficult to access. Make sure bathrooms and the kitchen have clear accesses. Too many accidents happen in these two areas to take chances. Check bed accesses as well. Dodging small tables, boxes, books etc. on the floor when leaving a bed at night in the dark is risky no matter what the age. Any work done here will be worth it to avoid ER trips and casts on broken bones.

Check stairs for railings. Install them if they are not there. Both sides are best if at all possible because having two hands holding on is generally better balance. Also, when carrying packages, either hand can be used.

Ramp If your relative is in a chair, a ramp may be necessary. This can be expensive and needs to be installed by a professional who has experience with ramps, the length, the incline degrees and the landing as well as the door opening. When a landing is too small, the person in the chair runs the risk of rolling backwards trying to make room for the swing of the door. Equally, if the ramp is too steep it is harder to navigate especially if the chair is not an electric one.

Ledges in doorways. These are a trip hazard especially if the lighting is poor. Reflective paint or tape is a good solution or even a simple bright color. If your relative is in a mobility chair these ledges in doorways can be very difficult to handle depending on how they have been installed. If there is no angle on each side (mini ramp) the chair has to hop over the obstacle. This is very jarring and, depending on such conditions as arthritis or osteoporosis, can be very painful.

Example: My father was in an electric wheelchair for the last few months of his life. He was very good at maneuvering his chair through doorways but there was one threshold in our new house that kept hanging his chair up so that he ended up jammed in the doorway.

Thankfully, all the doors in this house are 36 inches wide. However, he was a big man and a electric chair is quite heavy.

Even helping him out of the chair while my husband and I muscled the thing over the ledge was more than enough for us to call the builder and have a different threshold installed. The odd thing was this particular threshold was the same as all the rest and should have worked. There was a slight height difference in the way it fit to the floor on one side and that was the problem. No one had caught it because the issue was so tiny. Since then, I suggest to anyone who asks, check each ledge individually. Sometimes the problem is only visible when it is a problem.

Rugs and area carpets. Another trip hazard. Check the edges. Rolled ends or corners can catch on a foot, a cane or a walker. Double sided tape from a carpet store is one solution if the rug or carpet must stay. There is also non-skid material that can be put under the rug or carpet. I prefer to contact a professional who can access the situation and solutions based on products, climate and cost.

Check toilets. Most homes are equipped with standard toilets. These are too low for the average aging person to use. A new toilet isn't cheap nor is the professional to install it. However, falls happen very often in the bathroom. Depending on the injury, you could be looking at full time care temporarily or permanently as a result. A few hundred, difficult though it may be at the time, will save both of you a lot more in the long term.

Faucets Old, rusted or stiff faucets are difficult for aging hands. Mom or Dad may be so accustomed to them that they don't even notice the problem. Check each faucet. Even if it looks good it may not be, especially if your loved one has arthritis or osteoporosis. If you are reasonably handy, these can be changed by you. Knobs are harder on bone or muscle damaged hands. Handles are a good choice and, budget allowing, sensor faucets are available.

Install handrails in showers and beside toilets These grab bars can be very useful to the aging relative who has trouble sitting or standing or getting up from a sitting position. The devices need not be ugly. There are some attractive versions available. I would suggest that a professional be involved in the installation. These bars must bear weight and pull. Injury can result if the bar comes off the wall just as your loved one is off balance moving from position to another.

Doorknobs. If your loved one has arthritis, he/she may find it hard if not impossible to turn doorknobs. Consider changing out the knobs to handles. This, if you are reasonably handy, you can do yourself.

Check hot water heater temperature. As one ages, heat and cold sensitivity can change. Skin becomes fragile. Scalding is not unusual in the aging population. Changing the setting to a lower level can prevent a serious burn.

Check where the cookware is stored. Don't laugh. This may sound crazy, but most people tend to store the cookware down low and most of the pots and pans are heavy or awkward to handle. Try bending over with a walker or cane to wrestle that favorite big pot off the shelf it shares with three other pots nestled in it. Guess who wins that little battle? Find a way to get the cookware in a more easily assessable place.

Get a cart with rollers for shopping bags. Years ago, because I shopped in bulk, I had to haul fifteen to twenty bags of groceries into the house at a time. One day, I was annoyed enough to use my brain instead of my brawn. I had arrived home with the usual grocery suspects and more from the hardware store and the plant nursery. I had a cart in the garage for the outdoor stuff and I wheeled it to the trunk to unload. I felt like a fool as I stood there looking at about twenty bags of stuff, all that would have to be carried by hand in many, many trips, into the house. I grew a brain. I washed the cart and loaded it to overflowing and pushed it into the house and even to each place to unload. Shopping had never been so easy. I was thirty at the time. Every house I have had since has a cart for yard stuff and one for house stuff. I have passed this hint along to everyone I know. I've had laughs over the years but no one who tries it ever gives up his or her cart.

All of my relatives, living in their homes or mine, had their own cart. Even the ones with walkers were able to use the cart as long as the cart is strong enough and stable enough to be leaned on much as a person with a cane or walker will use a shopping cart in a store. Again, here I would consult a specialist about the safety issues of the cart you purchase. A medical equipment store may be able to advise you. Safety is paramount. If you doubt the stability of the cart do not provide one for your relative.

Lighting As your loved one ages; vision is often affected. In house lighting and even outdoor lighting can become a problem so subtly that often Mom or Dad doesn't even notice. Check those dark stairs that lead from the house to the yard, that closet that is a dark hole of storage with boxes on the top shelf that can topple down if not handled properly. What about that dark hallway that has no light? Each of these areas are places for falls, for bruising bumps into walls and corners. Many aging people are on blood thinners or an aspirin regiment that makes bruising a real issue. Battery operated lights, some are even motion sensitive are a solution here. Many types just stick to the wall. The local hardware store or the internet is a good source of products of varying prices. Outdoor lighting for pathways can be attractive as well as functional and earth friendly. There are solar lights available, again in a range of prices.

House Temperature Many of the aging population are more sensitive to hot or cold. Heaters need to be turned up in winter and fans or AC work harder in the summer. Power bills can become a real issue, especially on the limited retirement budget. Many power companies offer free assessments of appliances such as furnaces and AC units. Older equipment often means higher operating costs. There are also tax incentives offered for changing outdated appliances. This is not cheap by any means even with the various rebates and so forth. However, overloaded circuits are a fire hazard. Being too hot or cold to save money is also a health hazard. A person can die from either extreme.

There are many other possible changes that may need to be made, depending on living arrangements. Apartments are going to present different challenges than a stand-alone home, so I have tried to stay with the basics. The point is: try to get ahead of the emergency room trips. Life is a lot easier on everyone involved that way.

CHAPTER FOUR

COMING HOME TO LIVE WITH YOU

Let's talk about your loved one or ones coming to live with you. This trend is growing daily but it is not a new idea at all. Generational living has been around for centuries and is a way of life in many countries today. We, however, are coming back to it after a long break. Worse, we are coming back to it when families are struggling simply to identify themselves. Add to that issue, a single parent household or one in which both parents have to work, and time and resources become even more limited. Now add children and all the accompanying tasks and even less time and resources are available. Even if there are no children, even if it is simply one person trying to take on the responsibility of Mom or Dad or both, the situation is loaded with difficulties and potential disasters.

You've gotten that call or you have realized that Mom or Dad can't be alone any longer. They don't need a care facility, or they absolutely won't consider one. Okay, they can move in with you. You have an extra bedroom or two if the kids can double up. Mom will be closer. It will save travel time. You love Mom and you have always gotten along. Or maybe not. Dad is always trying to tell you what to do but you'll be at work most of the time, so it will be all right.

WRONG!!!! I wish I could tell you it is that easy, but it isn't. First, your loved one is used to his space. You are used to ruling your own life. BOTH OF THESE THINGS ARE GOING TO CHANGE.

All the love and caring in the world doesn't mitigate the demands of the lifestyle you are both entering. Love will soften the edges, but it won't change the physical needs or the financial ones. So, brace yourself. Life as you know it is over. Fighting that isn't going to get you anything but a stress headache and witch's own temper. Accept it. As hard as this sounds, it is the plain truth.

Deal with the facts. Start with the physical aspect of the move itself. Just popping Mom into the back bedroom isn't going to work. She is not a visitor and this not short term. She is losing her independence. She may be even considering herself a burden. Her home, one she has made and may have inhabited for years is no longer safe or useful. She can't take all of her things. These are just some of her thoughts, her fears, her frustrations. Here are some things to consider for you and her.

THE SIZE AND DÉCOR OF THE ROOM Mom has just left her house or apartment. She is going to have her own room in yours. Where is she going to put the things that matter to her. A favorite chair, a lamp, her bed, television? Her books or hobby? You've got this bedroom decorated to your taste. Is it hers? More than likely not, not in furniture or color.

I have had three different adults living in my home. My mother and father were the first. I sat down with them and discussed the things they wanted to bring with them. I already knew their style and color preferences, but I asked anyway. I can't say that I was actually thinking of my mother's choice. I was considering mine. She was a difficult woman in the best of moments, and this was not it. I figured the minute I got her, and my father moved in I would be told she hated the décor, and I would have to change it with her in residence. I was just getting ahead of the problem she could be.

As it happened, I learned that this basically self-motivated step reaped a reward for both of us. She felt very important right from the beginning because I had taken the time to ask and she did everything she could to cooperate as she thinned out her belongings to fit into the space.

WHERE IS THE BATHROOM? Many of the aging population are on blood pressure medicine or other medications that make middle of the night trips to the bathroom the norm. Having a bathroom down the hall or across the house can be disruptive especially if lights have to be turned on the make the trip. Try to pick a bedroom that is close to the bath your loved one is going to use. While we're in the bathroom, let's discuss the things necessary to make this a safe place for your relative.

BATHROOM MODIFICATIONS Handicap height toilets are higher off the floor than standard ones. Consider changing your existing water closet. I'm not sure why we even have the lower height anymore when the higher model is easier on the knees and more useable for most adults.

Install grab bars in the shower and around the toilet if your loved one needs assistance getting up or down. Also, tub/shower stalls are very difficult for the aging relative. Having to step over the tub and into a slick rounded tub bottom is a risk. An accident here probably means broken bones at best or death at worst. It is expensive to change but much better than the alternative if there is any way to stretch the budget.

If your loved one already needs help getting bathed or showered, consider one of the new walk-in tub/shower units that can be installed in most bathrooms. These can be expensive and definitely need a professional install. However, considering the budget and the long-term benefit may make it the answer to your situation.

KITCHEN PRIVILEGES First, find out from your Mom when she eats, how often and what she likes. You may think you know but you probably don't. If her schedule meshes with yours, GREAT. If not, the two of you need to decide on a schedule that works for you both. Is she cooking? Are you all right with her in your kitchen? Does she keep a neat workspace or a mess? All of this matters to both of you.

Ask questions. You can't work together if neither of you knows what the other thinks, wants or needs. If you are going to be cooking for your relative, is it going to be all three meals? If you are working, the answer is no unless you are going to make meals and put them in the refrigerator. This adds to your list. I have found this area to be one of the trickier areas to handle. My solution is to be actively involved as little as possible. I prefer to give my relatives as much freedom in this area as I can and to give them an option to avoid dealing with the early morning rush of getting my family off to the various locations of the day.

With a little planning, an area can be set up in your loved one's room for snacking or even making a drink at any hour. Mini frigs, some as small as a cube, can be set in place along with a coffee/tea maker, a toaster and even a small microwave. A sturdy bookshelf will hold the items and a small table will make a nice nook for eating, especially if placed by a window.

The focus here is to give your relative a place that is his, available 24/7 for that craving for a snack or just a cup of coffee without having to bother anyone or ask anyone's permission. The idea isn't to isolate your loved one as much as it is creating a home within a home where he can choose when to eat. This doesn't mean every meal unless that is his choice. Family meals can work well in this situation, making the food sharing time enjoyable rather than a ritual to endure. Example: My father liked to munch his way through the day rather than sit down to a meal. I do mean the day. He rarely slept, preferring naps so he was up and down all night. Having a place of his own, a mini kitchen of own meant the rest of us, those working could sleep like normal people and he could snack and watch TV whenever the mood struck.

I kept his frig stocked with his favorite drinks, sliced meats and produce for that late-night sandwich he loved, and his shelves loaded with his snack goodies. Paper plates, his idea, meant he just pitched his dishes in the trash, and I didn't even have to do clean up. It was a great arrangement for both of us.

When I suggested this idea to one of my friends, her one objection was the carpeting her mother's room. She had point. Accidents happen to us all, no matter what our age. If carpet is an issue, consider changing the flooring. I know it is expensive, but removal has side benefits. It is easier to keep the floors clean. A less expensive solution is to put a washable rug over the carpet. Make sure it is fastened down properly so as not to become a trip hazard.

The evening meal was generally shared by us all. My father, after my mother died, preferred to eat in front of his television so I would make a tray for him either from what I had cooked that night or something I had put up in the freezer. I tried not to be rigid on the menu at night, simply because I had found early on that evening meals for the aging persons in my families were often smaller and more snack like.

A freezer is invaluable here. I prefer making large quantities of things, parceling them up in meal size containers and freezing for future use. This frees up my time tremendously. However, this may not be time saving for everyone. Scan the freezer section of the supermarket, especially read labels if you have dietary issues to deal with in food selection. Organic meals are even available. I do use some of these to supplement my own creations as well. Cooking time can be minimized to fit your schedule. Also, with frozen meals, your loved one may cook his/her meal. He/she may even prefer to do so either regularly or occasionally. Be aware here of the sodium content of the prepared foods. Many of the aging population have restrictions in this area. Keep in mind that one meal may not be the daily intake. It may be multiples.

Another thing I made sure to have around in the kitchen is fruit, both canned and fresh. Maybe it is just the people I know or my friends but every one of us that is or has been taking care of relatives has noticed an increase in fruit intake.

PRIVACY Everyone, you included, needs alone time. Having a room in a busy home, with family, isn't conducive to privacy unless it is planned. If the room or rooms you have allotted to your relative has its own television, phone and small kitchen type area, you have gone a long way to maximizing the livability for you loved one and the privacy for both of you.

However, accidentally, I came up with an idea that added a touch for my parents in one of our homes. Depending on the style of the house or apartment, try putting a compression rod with a stylish curtain across the hall to close off your relative's area. Again, discuss this. The last thing you want is for them to feel shut out. This is their front door. They can pull it shut or leave it open. Their choice. Not yours.

Your relative can leave the bedroom in a robe or towel and head for the shower without worrying who might see them. The mother who doesn't feel well enough to put on her I-never-leave-my-room-without-it makeup can kick back in her favorite chair with a naked face and know that no one is going to find her indulging herself. Grandkids love visiting granddad who lives just down the hall. If the curtain is closed, you can hear them whispering about knocking.

NOISE If your loved one has a hearing issue, television, radio or music too loud becomes a real ear banging problem. Even though your relative may have hearing aids, wearing them may not be happening. Many find them irritating and prefer going without.

You, however, don't have a hearing deficit and don't want one. Closed caption is not always something that your relative likes or will use. Beyond that, it is only good for television. To save my hearing and my sanity, I found a device called an Easy Talk, there are others out there, but this one is very inexpensive and is similar to an iPod only the pod part is the size of a small phone.

My father found this to be his favorite hearing device. It had a volume dial and one ear bud attached to a tiny cord. The pod part popped into his shirt pocket. His thousands of dollars hearing aids stayed in his desk drawer and he used his Easy Talk all the time. No ear wax build up, no screeching in his ear on the phone and no lost conversations in the background. He could hear his favorite television shows and I didn't have to.

ENTRANCE Most homes and apartments don't have aging friendly entrances. Everything from steps and stairs to hills to climb in bad weather are common. Access your entrance. Even if your relative is fully mobile right now, he/she may not be in the future. Consider what you need to do to change things. Some changes are expensive and need a professional to modify. Some are relatively simple.

For steps and stairs, handrails are essential. Check the width of the steps and the height of the risers. The risers must be the same throughout the stair area. It is a real trip hazard for anyone if they are not. If your loved one is in a mobility chair of some kind, a ramp will need to be added. In a stand-alone house this is possible in most cases, design wise, but it is expensive. In an apartment, you will need to go through channels and that can be a lengthy process and often not successful in the way that you will want or need.

MAIL This may sound a little odd here but picking up the mail can end up being a bone of contention in your home. Mom or Dad are home most of the day, alone. The mail comes. Both of you are getting it delivered to the same address. Dad picks up the letters and bills. Pulls his stuff out and lays yours somewhere today and someplace different tomorrow. He can't remember or you just like going through your own mail first or don't want him knowing you got a bill from that company for something you bought he didn't think you should. The problems aren't much one at a time but over months and years of comments and migrating mail, you may end up wishing you hadn't skipped this step.

If you work, one solution would be to get a post office box close to your job or home. His mail goes to the house and yours gets handled by you. Or, if Dad stills drives, he might be the one happier with a post office box. It gives him a chance to pop to the post office, stop off for coffee at his favorite hang out and talk to his friends. Or, you may be able to arrange with the post person to have the two occupants bundled separately in the same box. Dad takes his bundle and leaves yours.

IF AT ALL POSSIBLE, CREATE THIS NEW HOME WITHIN A HOME ON THE GROUND FLOOR Whether your loved one needs the ground floor accommodations or not at this point, there is a strong chance that as aging continues climbing stairs, indoors or out, will be an issue.

Mobility aids are great on reasonably flat surfaces but add stairs and, in the case of the outdoors, inclement weather and your relative will be safer with a companion as he negotiates stairs. Even ramps can be an issue unless the ramp has been weather proofed according to your climate.

Indoors, the stairs can be even more of an issue depending on how old the house is. Walkers do not fit completely on stairs. It is up to the person needing this device to balance it on each stair. Try it yourself and you will see the problem. It's tiring for one thing. By the time you get to the top you have had a workout just lifting the walker, balancing without it as you place it on the next step. Going down is an accident waiting to happen as mom leans forward to put the walker on each step below.

If you decide to skip the walker and be mom's balancing point, you either have to take the device to the top of the stairs for her, then walk down and walk her back up or reverse the process. How many times a day? What if you aren't there?

Or you can buy an upstairs walker and a downstairs one. Take your wallet.

Most insurances won't pay for two walking aid devices of any kind.

RETRO FIT YOUR HOME This is expensive even if you are doing small things such as changing doorknobs to handles. Add stairs that need to be made accessible for someone with mobility issues, handicap (I really wish someone would come up with a better description) height toilets and wider door openings and you could have bought a luxury car.

I haven't found an insurance that covers any retro fitting. That doesn't mean there isn't one out there. Research this avenue just in case. However, you may find that there are organizations or churches that do offer financial help. Our church and our pastor obtain materials and provide labor to put in such things as ramps at no cost to the recipient. Check these sources in your area and if you do have them and can volunteer even a few hours every now then you would be helping someone who really needs it.

CHOOSE A HOME FOR YOUSELF THAT WILL ACCOMMODATE THE NEEDS OF YOUR AGE-RELATED FAMILY. This solution isn't right for everyone. I am not suggesting that you sell your home and buy another. But if you are in the process of moving consider the possible future needs of any relative for whom you may be caring in the future. Consider yourself as well if you plan to make this new home the one in which you age.

Most homes in the past and currently DO NOT ALLOW FOR AGING CHANGES. Think about where you live now. On the basis of what you have been reading, how would it stack up? How wide are the interior doors? How aging friendly are the stairs? How high off the floor are the toilets? Is there only a tub shower with a huge edge you have to step over into a rounded bottom where someone, even you, could slip and fall?

If you are looking around your home and thinking it doesn't matter, read again. It does.

Since you are in a moving mood, add some things to your wish list besides granite counter tops and an open concept. By the way, this last one is a trend right now that I hope continues because it is aging friendly. There are few doorways to contend with and, depending on furniture placement, it means as the needs grow the couch and chairs can be easily moved or decreased.

If possible, find a place with an in-law suite. This usually consists of a bedroom, often more generously sized than the average, and a bath. If the bath needs retro fitting for aging, consult a contractor for costs. If you are purchasing, figure the cost into the price of the house. Some choices will be more expensive than others. If you are renting, you will naturally need the landlord's permission to make any changes unless he is willing to pay himself. Unlikely but you won't know if you don't ask. Cost share may be possible. Again, you won't know if you don't ask.

As you can see there is more to being a caregiver, than is first apparent. Your surroundings matter a great deal. The people with whom you are sharing your home are important and you and they deserve the best environment you can provide. The suggestions I have given are just that suggestions. Hopefully, they will help you ease the stress and the labor of this new lifestyle. But, as with everything, you don't have to address all these issues at once unless the one for whom you are caring needs each thing. If that is the case, it is important that you get financial assistance unless you have a really deep wallet. Most of us don't. I will be discussing this aspect of your situation in a later chapter. There is help out there but, depending on your state, it isn't always easy to find, and I haven't discovered any one source that will cover everything. However, in this situation, any help makes a huge difference.

CHAPTER FIVE

BUILDING A HOUSE

This chapter is not going to apply to most care givers however, there will be some. At this writing, four years ago, I designed and had built a house that was aging friendly. It didn't break the budget and it doesn't look at all like what you would expect. I built it for myself, my father and my husband. My father already lived with me and I used the design of the mother-in- law suite that he had built in the house I had bought from him as a basis for the new house. His version lacked storage and covered parking. It also lacked its own washer/dryer and AC unit.

Because my husband and I were retiring and moving to a different part of the state, I decided to create a home using the experience I had gleaned in the forty odd years of care giving. I am no more eager to leave my home than most people. Equally, I don't want to live with my daughters. They have their own lives and personalities and I know what care giving demands of the care giver.

Pencil in hand, after multiple trips through model homes to find a basic design I liked and could tweak, I started measuring and drawing. The result is a one-story house with entrances at ground level. On one third of the house pad, the ground was raised to achieve this. Every window but one has a view outdoors even if I am laying bed or sitting in a chair. All of us love the outdoors and didn't want to lose the ability to see out if any of us was sick in bed or just didn't feel like getting up one day. Having lived in a number of houses through the years I knew that windows often weren't really offering a view unless I was standing.

Equally, we wanted to be outside on even inclement days. A porch was a necessity here. So, there is a wide screened porch with rocking chairs over-looking a small waterfall and pond surrounded by an open-air patio. Water gardens have always been a bit of hobby, so, with the help of crew of friends, we dug and planted and hauled rocks until the garden was complete. It is not only restful but filled with the memories of the laughter and the sweat of its creation.

My father's apartment shares the porch and the view. He has his own kitchen as do I. He also has his own garage, phone and television. His alarms for smoke, fire and carbon monoxide are hooked to mine. If his are set off so are mine. All toilets in both houses are handicap height and the main showers in both areas have no ledges so entering requires no stepping over tub rims. It is even possible, if necessary, to drive a wheelchair straight into the shower itself for transfer to the shower seat. I do have a Jacuzzi tub, but the surround is extra wide so all I have to do is sit on the edge and then swing my legs over into the tub. The faucets are offset to one end making entry that much easier.

The flooring in either house is tile or wood. My father wanted carpet in the main room of his apartment. The pad is thinner than most because, at first, he was using a walker and a cane. The thicker pad makes both a little more difficult.

We both have tankless hot water heaters to prevent the lack of hot water when all of us may have be running the washer or taking showers at the same time. All counter tops are thirty-six inches as are all doorways, making both much more usable with a wheelchair which ended up being a fact of both my husband's and my father's life. There are no doorknobs, only handles. Both areas are open concept which makes both appear huge when in reality neither really is. My father's apartment is 25' x 35' and that includes a garage. My own, which is a three-bedroom, two baths is approximately 35' x 57'. To date the only comments, I get on the house are not based on how aging friendly it is. No one even notices the mobility impaired adjustments.

Despite all these tweaks to the construction process, for the square footage of the house within a house, my home is considerably less expensive than most of the same size. There was no downgrade in quality of workmanship or materials either. It took planning and it took attention to what I wanted in details. I don't care for granite or quartz counters. Drop a lid on the stone surface and my ears seem to ring forever. Plus, granite needs sealing and maintenance, something I did not want to add to my list as I aged. I didn't want crown molding either. However, I did want bamboo flooring and tile. Ten-foot-high ceilings were another must along with ceiling fans and custom cabinets.

In short, with planning and keeping in mind what you like and want and your budget you can build a home to accommodate any care giving you may be currently doing or any you may do in the future. You may also, if you decide this is your last home, build this new house with your own aging in mind. Professional help is worth the cost depending on your circumstances or you can research the various requirements for impaired living arrangements and consider what may be your needs in the future. If you absolutely love wide sweeping stairs, have them but build the stair well walls with the idea of adding a chair lift if you ever need one. Then should the need arise, you will have the plans and the proper support in the walls so installation will be much easier and much less expensive than it would have been without your forethought. Thought here in the construction process makes your aging a phase of life that under most conditions won't require you giving up a home you love.

Many of my relatives and those of friends have had to leave their houses not because of the aging process but because the house itself was not set up to accommodate the changing needs of the owner. Often the cost to retro fit this kind of home is so prohibitive than moving is the only option. Homes are so intensely personal, especially ones that have hundreds of memories of a lifetime of use that just moving is heart wrenching. The new place never seems to be the same and there is always that memory of the home that you couldn't keep because you got too old or infirmed. To make a choice because you want to is one thing. To make a choice because you have to is something none of us wants or ever really accepts.

CHAPTER SIX

NEEDS OF THE CARE GIVER

We have talked about the physical needs of the move but not the emotional ones. In the sheer volume of work needed to combine households—make no mistake that is what you are doing here—it is easy to forget or simply not think about what you are doing. When one person taking in one person is the case, dealing with the emotional demands as they crop up is fairly straightforward.

If your situation is a family, single parent, two parents, blended families, this becomes a minefield that seems to never stop blowing up in your face. If you have a job plus any of these situations the problems are mind boggling. Here are some ideas for approaching this minefield. Again, the idea here is do your best. You won't eliminate the explosions but, hopefully, you will reduce or contain them. Remember, you want and need this new arrangement to work, for your loved one, yourself and those for whom you already care.

BLENDED FAMILIES This family group may be constant, or it may be fluctuating on a weekly or monthly basis. Mom and Dad are married but each brought children to the home. One group stays and the other comes for regular visits. Now, Mom's dad is going to be living with the couple. He is blood kin to half the children and not the other half. The husband didn't start out with this man as his father-in-law and now he is sharing his home with his wife's father.

Are you getting a headache yet? I'm not trying to play counselor here. I'm not qualified. What I am saying is, don't get so caught up in the move that you forget the people involved. Talk to your partner. Talk to the children. Talk to your partner's children together and separately. Explain, age appropriately, the situation and what it will mean to you, to them and to your partner. Listen to their responses with an open mind. You cannot deal with a problem if you don't know it exists. Depending on the issue, a support group or counseling may be needed. Above all don't ignore the issues thinking any or all will go away. How often does that happen in real life?

A COUPLE Just because someone loves you doesn't mean that person loves your relatives. Now, you are saying that relative or parents is moving in with the two of you. You've probably outlined all the reasons for the move, but have you simply asked if your partner is on board with your choice? Over the years, I have found this one simple thing is often overlooked by those I talked to in similar situations.

When my husband and I got married, we both had families, mother and father. His were very aged already and I was only nineteen and he was twenty- three. We both loved our parents and we both knew that if either pair ever needed help, we were probably going to be the ones who would be giving it. Between us, we decided that he would decide what was best for his and I would support him, and I would decide for mine and he would support me.

The simplicity of youth sometimes is better than the complexity of maturity. It was in our case. I grew to love his parents, but their care was time consuming and inconvenient as they stayed in their home until his mother's death. His father remarried a year and a half later and we had two to take care of instead of one and that new person was a complete unknown to us. When David's father died, his third wife's family took her home with them.

My parents came to live with us. My husband didn't have the same kind of relationship with them that I had enjoyed with his and yet we shared the same house and stayed married for twenty more years. In both cases, we talked to each other, good and bad.

Through the years and the people who have asked how we did it, often those in similar situations that weren't working well, I found that one of the biggest issues was neither partner talked honestly with the other nor listened if a dialogue had been opened. I know this hard for many. Who wants to admit to being discouraged, angry or just plain defeated by the demands of this new life? Few of us. Try. For your sake. For your partner's sake. Even if the partner can't help with the day to day physical demands, sometimes just having an ear is enough.

If you have children, the issue becomes even more complex. Having Mom, Dad or both in the house means that everyone in the family isn't going to get as much attention as he/she had. Again, talk to the children, age appropriately, and discuss the changes you're making. Involve them if possible. Caring for others is important to anyone's development. Respect, interest empathy and sympathy all come into the picture. Let the children help, be a part of what you are doing.

You have a choice. Make this new lifestyle an enriching experience or a burden.

SINGLE PARENT As a single parent you are already doing two jobs, mom and dad. Now you are going to be adding one or more people into your home. In some cases, this can be a very good thing. Combined incomes help both of you. Having someone always in the house means that when your child is ill or home from school for whatever reason you don't have to worry with day care or a babysitter or taking time off work. For the one living with you this also means that they can see themselves helping you. Instead of being a burden, he/she feels important, even necessary.

However, all parties need to talk to each other, understand what is changing and what is not. Again, the key here is listening and working out as many problems as possible from the beginning. You won't get them all but you will be setting up a format that lets everyone understand that you will be listening when they speak and you will try to work out a way to make whatever the issue is better.

Now, let's talk about the physical demands on your time. If you work in the home or out, the demands exist either way. I have lived both sides of this picture and I personally found the work-out-of-the-home trickier to handle.

When I worked off site, I found I only had to arrange my days off to have at least one in the middle of the week and I could schedule the various errands and doctor appointments around those days. That did not account for emergencies but those, thankfully, were few and I had employers that understood the problem and were flexible with the situation. I simply made up lost time. If you can't work things out, especially in a crisis, the Family Medical and Leave Act may be an option.

Every employer is different, and today's workplace contains pressures that can make any of us think twice or maybe ten times about this next step. Only you will know what is best. However, if possible, talk to your employer. Explain your current situation, include any possible crisis points that you may know. Have a plan of action that you can offer as to how you will handle the demands of your personal life and still maintain the standard of your job performance. Most employers will appreciate the efforts you are making both in your personal life and your professional one.

WORKING FROM HOME ONE OR MORE DAYS A WEEK MAY BE AN OPTION. THIS OPTION GENERALLY APPLIES TO OFFICE TYPE JOBS. There are all kinds of names for this kind of arrangement, virtual office, remote office, telecommunicating. The premise is simple. You have an office set up in your home and handle your professional work from there. Utilities, such as internet lines, phones and possibly even electric usage are sometimes paid for by the company in this type of setting.

Keep in mind, you are going to need quiet, space and time to make this set up work effectively. This means talking to any members of the household who are present during these work hours. Screaming children in the background when you are on an important real time computer hook up is not a good image.

FLEXIBLE HOURS MAY BE ANOTHER. Simply, this is working a few hours a certain number of days a week and the rest working longer to make up the time needed for a full work week. This solution needs planning. It's not as easy as it sounds. The long days increase fatigue and even if the next day is short it rarely feels that way as you try to squeeze in every task you have to do. If at all possible, involve your family in some of the chores, if not in the care giving, in the meals for all of you, laundry etc. You need help. Ask for it.

WORKING PART TIME OR AS A CONSULTANT ON A JOB TO JOB BASIS MAY ACTUALLY BE COST EFFECTIVE FOR YOU. This solution could even involve your current employer. If it is a solution both of you have discussed, a little time and number crunching here may go a long way in helping you to make an informed decision. Often, the time spent working is expensive, travel costs, clothing, spending money etc. just to name a few. The benefit here with the reduced hours may be more than just the physical and mental demands.

DEPENDING ON YOUR FAMILY SITUATION AND BUDGET, CONSIDER BEING PAID TO DO THE CARE GIVING. This sounds mercenary I know but, if you are working, generally you need the money, for your living expenses, your children etc.

Example: Maybe there are multiple family members but none as close as you. You're the one risking your job, your career for this new lifestyle. Talk to your relatives, discuss being a paid care giver. If this choice works for all of you handle it as you would any other work. Get it in writing. The internet offers a number of sites with printable contracts. Or you can contact a lawyer for professional help. Above all, stand firm about making this kind of arrangement a business one. Life happens. Family dynamics change. Having a contract protects all parties much better than not having one. Spell out the terms. Remember, this now means you are self-employed. There are tax benefits and tax responsibilities attached to this choice. Research both so that you and the IRS don't have a problem in the months and years to come.

FINALLY, DEPENDING ON THE SITUATION OF YOUR LOVED ONE, YOU MAY NEED TO CONSIDER TAKING A LEAVE OF ABSENCE. In today's work environment, this can be a risky and scary step for many to consider. The leave may be one that is short term in nature, such as your loved one is recovering from surgery or hospitalization for some illness. However, if a long-term absence is on the table, most companies have guidelines if it is allowed at all.

This option, unlike the others listed, does not include a regular paycheck. You are on your own. As critical as the situation is that has made you consider this solution, be sure that you can sustain it for longer than you envision. There are no reliable timetables that I have found in care giving nor has there been for anyone I know. Days often turn into weeks and weeks to months. Losing a job on top of the crisis that required the absence is not a situation you want to face. If at all possible, find another way.

Now, let's discuss working out of your home. This is my personal favorite and where I have spent most of my working life. As great as it sounds to most people, in reality there are number of challenges that occasionally make me wish I had never set up a home office nor kept one active for thirty years.

SPACE is the first issue. It isn't just the square footage needed. It's privacy on which you can depend. If you're going to be on the phone or on the computer web cam, you will need privacy and silence in the background. You will also need storage and hook ups for your equipment. Having any or all of these three spread all over the home, means time lost looking for stuff and arguments when other family members don't respect your working hours.

GET AT LEAST THE SKELETON EQUIPMENT TO SET UP YOUR WORKSPACE. Everyone has a budget. However, setting up your office or work area is a necessity. The more you have to make do or look for things the more hours you use that could have been used for something else. The idea here is to make your life as easy as possible where you can. There is enough you cannot change.

MAKE A LIST OF RULES FOR WORKING TIME. I am a writer and prefer to work in the morning when I am fresh, usually from eight until noon. About the second year, after a number of unnecessary interruptions, I finally learned a valuable lesson. Make a rule and stick to it no matter how much you love the person trying to get around it.

DON'T INTERRUPT UNLESS THE EMTs ARE ON THE WAY! Was my battle cry.

I sat down with my parents and discussed my work hours. I usually saw them early each day, around six am. We went over the schedule for that day then I went off to work. I also sat down with my family and discussed this clearly. Every member of the household tested this edict. Being firm was hard but necessary. There were no exceptions. Make one and you will never have peace again in my experience, especially if a child or demanding relative is involved.

MAKE A CALENDAR OF EVENTS FOR THE HOUSEHOLD. To this day, when I no longer have anyone to care for, I have a calendar on my desk. You can also create a calendar on the computer. The point is, do yourself a favor and make one. Every event, appointment, phone call or chore is on the thing. It's a record and a reminder. If I need to know when I talked to someone it is there. If I need to know when I have my next massage it is there. If I need to know when to change the alarm batteries it is there.

No, this is not compulsive as much as a survival skill. I have run as many as three different generations, multiple people in each out of my home. Try doing that and keeping your sanity without a list somewhere just to remind you to feed the dog.

EVERYONE NEEDS A DAY OFF. Take a day off weekly. You need to recharge even if you think you are a super powered person. Yes, there will certain things you have to do on that day but otherwise, please yourself. Go to the mall, eat out at a special place, curl up with a book and tell everyone to pretend you aren't there. Play, relax and just enjoy not having to do something for someone else.

If at all possible, get someone, a family member or a friend, to come and watch over your relative while you escape. By the way, leave the guilt at home on this one. Depending on how long you have gone without having a day off, this might be harder than it sounds, and you may be resistant to the idea as well. 'How can I go, Mom needs me?'

Yes, she does and that is the very reason you need a break. You are carrying a heavy load. Been there. Done that. Ask any care giver. We all feel guilt. It is impossible not to feel it. We all want to be there every minute, but we also wish we didn't have to do this. No matter how much you care, there are days and will continue to be days when you just want to walk away. It hurts. You're tired. You just want some peace. There is a pressure cooker of emotions boiling away here and it needs to be released if only for a little while. TAKE THE BREAK! When you come back, you will feel better and the more often you let yourself relax the better you will be able to handle the demands of loving and care giving.

Now, let's address the stay at home man or woman. Generally, when this occurs there are children involved. No matter what the age, a child is work. As an infant, it's bottles, diapers and potty training to name just a few. School age, it is trips to everywhere under the sun and a few you have never considered. It isn't uncommon to feel as though you live in your car. Meanwhile, mom or dad or both need doctor appointments or shopping trips. Cleaning and washing for them as well your household may be in the mix as well.

Without a list of some kind that scenario is chaos. Kids whining about the cupcakes you forgot to make for school and mom wondering if you forgot she was supposed to have her hair done won't be an exception they will be the headache, high blood pressure producing everyday occurrence.

Parenting is a job, a profession, a vocation and an avocation. And it is care giving. When you add another generation into the mix of the existing household guess who is going to bear the brunt of the workload? You!

SET UP SOME RULES, SOME GUIDELINES FOR EVERYONE INVOLVED. Everyone is going to be giving up something in time and attention. You are only one person. Make your minutes and your hours count because when any of those for whom you care don't get what he/she thinks he deserves; you are going to hear about it.

PARCEL OUT CHORES. Everyone is capable of contributing. Let them. Everyone gains when they participate in the home you all share. Mom may not have the energy she once had but maybe she can read bedtime stories or sit in the yard or park and watch the children play. Dad can't build like he used to, but he may be able to oversee the science project your daughter is making. The kids might not be old enough to run the laundry, but they can unload the dryer and pull their own clothes out of the load and put them away. Your partner can handle a few errands on the way home from work.

Just because you don't have a traditionally defined job doesn't mean you aren't working. Every woman I know who has worked on both sides of this coin feels that being at home is a great deal more labor intensive than being on a traditional job.

Keep in mind that every home situation is different. Co-operation is not always the dynamic that runs your family. If you have a difficult relative to bring into your home or for whom you care out of the home, you will find that having easy days is an exception rather than the rule. When you add the demands of your existing home life, the problems mount. Be realistic about what you can and can't do. Be firm with those around you and even with other family members. You know the ones who are quick with advice and least in sight when you need help. Remind everyone, if necessary, that you are carrying a great deal. If the care giver ends up needing a care giver, who is going to take your person who needs a care giver??? Try to arrange time for your relative that is someone else's responsibility besides yours. Mom visiting your sister for a day is a good example or your brother taking Dad on a fishing trip for the weekend. You get a mini vacation and your loved one gets an outing with another part of the family. As a care giver, it is easy for everyone to take for granted what you do and that includes you. Sharing the load is good for everyone, you and those for whom you care.

CHAPTER SEVEN

PAPERWORK, PAPERWORK

This part of the care giving process is very irritating and boring for some of us. It's very intrusive for others. And for most us, it is a sensitive subject on our good days. Sorry, but it needs to be done. You can't help your loved one if you don't know the full extent of his needs. You need to know about things such as insurance and bill paying because, if your relative has a crisis, he may not be able to tell you how to keep his personal life in order until he is well again. You can't make decisions if you don't know where the paperwork is to implement those decisions.

Sit down with your relative and explain why you need to know. Please, don't force agreement onto your loved one. Circumstances permitting, allow your relative time to adjust to the fact that he/she needs to share this for both your sakes.

I am listing things that I have found most helpful and the reasons why each matter. I am also grouping these things in, what I consider, order of importance. Some are obvious, some are not. This list may not constitute a complete group in your case. So add, at will, the extras. In a crisis, having the paperwork can make a big difference. I will be addressing many of these issues individually in the coming chapters.

THE WILL. Know who the executor is, especially if it is not you. Make sure the will is current and exactly what your loved one wants now, especially if that loved one has recently lost a spouse or partner. The heir situation may have completely changed. If this is the case, help your relative have a new will draw up as soon as possible. Keep a copy of the will in a safe place. I also kept another copy in a bag I kept for trips to the hospital (this will be discussed in depth shortly).

PENSION CHECKS DUE. Social Security is probably applicable here. Pensions from employment, disability or military may also be part of your loved one's income. Work with your relative here. His ability to be open with you depends on his personality. If he/she feels he is still capable there is every chance your relative will refuse outright to discuss this aspect with you.

Example 1: My father, an extremely independent man, was completely capable of handling his finances up until the day he died. He didn't need me to handle this area for him. However, because it is always possible, even for the very young, to have an accident or illness that incapacitates for a time, we discussed what his bills were in general terms and where I could find his paperwork if the need arose. He made a master list for me, dates his moneys were direct deposited in his bank account and his bills, phone, car payment, insurance, car tag, car insurance etc. He put the list where he always kept his bill book. All I had to do was open a drawer and I had everything I needed to handle his affairs. I did not need to know the amounts of anything for this list to work in a crisis. This way of handling the situation was a good compromise for us but certainly not the only way of doing finances.

Example 2: A friend of mine, a woman in her early seventies has all of her information with a company which has created software for safe and secure cloud storage. This program allows my friend to choose to whom she gives access to her information, for how long and she can track, at any time, who has done what with what in her files. Her children all live in other states. Although they are close emotionally, obviously they are not geographically. This physical distance is a major problem in a crisis situation. This program allows my friend's daughter to access any document (assuming my friend has allowed it) to fax to a hospital or doctor in the case of emergency or to handle any bill remotely until my friend is well enough to do it herself.

Again, this is not the only way to handle this problem. The point is the financial aspect must be addressed. Pretending it isn't there can cause big problems.

MEDICAL INFORMATION Get a list of all of your loved one's doctors. This should include addresses and phone numbers. Make a calendar of all appointments even if your loved one is still driving and usually goes to the doctor alone. I have always kept two, one for me and one for my relative.

Even though your relative is independent, this may not always be the case. If you know your relative is scheduled for a visit that day you will be in a better position to rearrange your own schedule to accommodate his. Also, if you should get a phone call from the doctor's office telling you that your loved one is being admitted to the hospital and you need to come get him, you won't be wondering where exactly the doctor is.

Believe it or not, I had this happen once. The person was new and really upset. She didn't even get the doctor's name out. With caller ID I could call back but what if I hadn't had it? Time would be lost, and my father would have been at risk while the office figured out that I wasn't there. Obviously, this was a mistake, but they do happen and often when someone can least afford it.

INSURANCE Chances are your relative is on Medicare or Medicaid if there is a disability involved. Private insurance either as a supplement or replacement may or may not apply depending on finances. You will need copies of the insurance cards. No hospital or doctor I have ever had contact with will treat without these two things and a picture ID, usually a driver's license.

Every relative I have cared for, carried his Medicare card and supplemental insurance card and driver's license in his wallet. I kept a copy of each with me as well. I can't tell you how many times we either got separated or one of them forgot his wallet. Having my copy with me saved my relative from waiting for treatment while I went home for a copy.

MEDICATIONS Most doctors and hospitals ask you to bring your medications with you rather than a list. In the case of the doctors, this is relatively simple but with a hospital it becomes problematic. Hospitals do not typically allow a patient to use his/her medications. The bottles can't be left unattended while you deal with your loved one and the hospital won't keep them safe for you. If there are a lot of medications, I've had as many as fifteen different prescriptions at times, you can see the problem.

I make a computer-generated list and keep it updated every time my relative gets a new prescription or a change in dosage. I don't just copy the drug name and dosage but the whole label of each bottle, including prescription number, pharmacy and pharmacy phone number. I have found only one hospital that needed this. A simple call to the pharmacy to verify the dosage was easy and fast because all of the information on the bottle was there.

It is critical to keep this list updated. If in doubt, take the drugs with you and deal with the handling issue on site. Doctors and the medical staff need to know what your loved one is taking, how much and how often.

I also like to have a list of when the drugs are taken. Don't count on the bottle here. Ask your relative when each pill is taken. Blood pressure medications, diabetes drugs and others are being used to control conditions that require monitoring. If a level is off, the doctor needs accurate information to adjust the dosage. If you report your loved one just took the drug when in reality, he took his pills four hours before, the doctor is not going to be able to accurately adjust the medication level for optimum results.

POWER OF ATTORNEY If your loved one is hospitalized, especially with no warning, it is going to be up to you to handle their affairs as seamlessly as possible. Hopefully, you have had a discussion with your loved one and have a complete idea of what bills exist and when payment is due.

A power of attorney can be used to cover this contingency. Depending on the length of stay, usually a phone call and a fax is all that is required to allow you to discharge your relative's responsibilities until he/she is well enough to handle them. It is possible your relative won't feel comfortable with this as it gives you the right to take over his/her affairs. Taking the time to discuss what a power of attorney actually means, and the conditions involved when it could be used may help allay concerns. If it doesn't, depending on the reason why it doesn't, there are other ways to handle the situation.

Example: My husband found his father was more comfortable simply adding my husband's name to all his accounts, including signing his house to his son in his lifetime. When he died, his foresight and trust in my husband made the settling of his estate considerably easier than it would have been. This is not a solution for either side with which everyone can be comfortable.

Another possibility is to have a joint account at the bank. This allows bill paying and so forth by either of you. This solution won't address more complicated matters but is better than no plan at all. There can be complications that can arise in which accounts can be frozen if prior arrangements haven't been made.

As hard as it is to face, hospitalization for your loved one is very probable, and life won't stop when it happens. Neither you nor he/she needs the added stress of unpaid bills or financial entanglements that can be easily avoided with a little forethought.

And, if this is the time that your loved one can't come home again, having at least some of the paperwork in place will help you handle his/her affairs in the best possible way for both of you. Closing out an estate, no matter what the size is time consuming and demanding when you will already be tired, stressed and grieving. Having been involved with or handled alone, more than one of these situation, I can say I have silently and sometimes, not so silently thanked each of those whom I loved for their trust and their choices in this every day matter that can be such a minefield.

CHAPTER EIGHT

INSURANCE

I know, the last thing you want to discuss is insurance. Few people have anything good to say about the subject and almost everyone has, at least, one horror story. However, if you are care giving or going to be care giving, you will be dealing with insurance.

There are a few constants.

•COVERAGE CHANGES CONSTANTLY.

•COVERAGE CHANGES FROM COMPANY TO COMPANY.

•COVERAGE CHANGES FROM YEAR TO YEAR.

•COVERAGE CHANGES IN DEDUCTIBLES AND PREMIUMS (IN THE CASE OF PRIVATE).

•COVERAGE CHANGES WITH GOVERNMENT ADMINISTRATION.

Because coverage changes constantly, it is necessary to ask questions, to understand what your policy does and does not do, what Medicare covers, and it does not cover and what your costs will be. I am not addressing this subject just from the viewpoint of a consumer. I worked with insurance in a doctor's office. I had to train myself, so I didn't have anyone to tell me an in-house procedure. I made my own and along the way I discovered simple ways to deal with insurance. Some were methods I had always used. Some are methods I developed trying to get bills paid so that I didn't have to rebill the patient. None of this makes me an expert. I don't think anyone can be. Every company has a different way of explaining benefits. A few of the terms are the same but that's about it. Even people in the business have to research plans, groups and so forth. Worse, what is true one day is not the next.

The stakes in this insurance game are extraordinarily high. First, and most important of all, is your health and your life. Mistakes with insurance can leave you paying for treatments you can't afford. Choosing whether to buy groceries or medicines is all too common in this country. When facing hundreds of thousands of dollars in doctor or hospital costs, declaring bankruptcy can seem the only way to survive. This is a terrible commentary on insurance in general. However, until there is a better way, you will be dealing with all these risks. Research is a good way to help stack the odds a little better your way.

Before we begin, let's define simply what some of the insurance words mean. The ones I've chosen are the money words. All the rhetoric in the world doesn't matter to me if I can't see the bottom line. These are the words that make up the bottom line, the amount you owe or don't owe.

DEDUCTIBLE This is a lump sum amount that the insurance company will cover but will not pay on your claims every year. The insurance company requires you to pay a certain amount of allowed charges before they will begin paying on your claim. For instance, Medicare Part B requires you to pay $198 deductible for 2020.

Example: You go to the doctor on January 2 for a regular visit. He charges $75 for that visit to all his patients but he participates with Medicare which only allows $50 for that service. The patient will have to pay the full $50 to the doctor's office for that day. The next day the patient goes for a chest X-Ray that the doctor ordered at an imaging center. They charge $300 for that service and they participate with Medicare which allows $200, ($200-$50=$150 – The patient will have to pay ($198-50 =$148) Medicare will pay 80% of the remaining $2.00 and the patient will owe a total of $148.40).

OUT OF POCKET – Is generally an amount owed by the patient until it is reached then the insurance will begin to pay their claims at 100% (less copays due) on remaining services for that year. Also known as a Catastrophic Cap if you have Tricare coverage.

Example: The patient has an 80/20 policy with a $500 annual deductible and $5000 Out-of-Pocket Limit. That means he/she will pay up to $5500/year in Medical expenses before their insurance will begin paying claims at 100%. This is true no matter what kind of overage they have (PPO/EPO/Commercial) -The patient is admitted to the hospital for 6 days for a procedure and recovery time. The total bill is $100,000 but the hospital participates with that insurance plan and agrees to accept their contract rate. For this procedure they agree to allow $50,000. Now the patient automatically owes $500 before admission because he has no other claims for the year. Then the insurance will pay 80% of the next $25,000 and then 100% of the remaining $24,500. Finally, the patient will owe a total of $5,500 for that hospital stay and nothing else for the rest of the year.

CO-PAY -Copays are set amounts that are due by the patient prior to services being rendered in all medical facilities and doctors' offices except emergency room visits. ER visits the patient must be accessed and treatment begun before the copay can be asked for by the hospital personnel. Copays are due all year long regardless of the patient meeting their deductibles and costshare limits. Generally, they are fairly small but can add up quickly like in the case of physical therapy which requires lots of visits during a 4 to 6 weeks treatment plan. Or for hospital admissions that charge a couple hundred dollars per day copays.

BILLED TO YOU This amount will appear on some kind of statement sent to you when both primary and secondary (if you have one) have paid. This amount is your responsibility. Depending on the amount and your circumstances this dollar figure can usually be paid in installments. You will need to contact the provider to make payment arrangements other than 'payment in full'. If you can only afford a very small amount per month you will have to support that need with documentation. The proof required varies with the business involved. There are some agencies available to help in these cases which will be discussed in another chapter.

There are many more terms involved in the insurance industry but these four are the basic money words. This part focuses on the insurance itself.

MEDICAID is insurance for those who cannot afford it, mostly only children, pregnant women and senior citizens can qualify for coverage. It is administered by the state the patient lives in.

MEDICARE is offered by the Federal government. At the moment, not all Medicare benefits start at sixty-five. The age for this is increasing. If you don't already know your age to receive Medicare, a simple phone call or checking on the internet will give it to you. You can qualify for Medicare early if you have End Stage Renal Disease or are permanently disabled. Check with the Medicare website for more information.

Assuming you do have Medicare, your benefits, in general, for medical care are 80% of the allowed contract cost.

An example of what this means to you is: The doctor charges $3000 for a certain procedure. He has a contract with Medicare, in other words he accepts Medicare patients in his office. Medicare allows $2000 for this procedure. There is already $1000 dollar difference. DON'T START SCREAMING YET. The doctor will be paid 80% of the $2000 allowed cost which is $1600. Assuming you have met your deductible for the year, your cost will only be $400 ($2000 - $1600 = $400). You should not be billed $1400 ($3000 - $1600 = $1400). If a doctor becomes a provider for an insurance, Medicare, Medicaid or private, he is signing a contract with that company that allows him to charge the patient only so much for each service.

THE DOCTOR CAN NOT PASS THE DIFFERENCE BETWEEN HIS CHARGES AND THE CONTRACT PRICE ON TO YOU. He can certainly pass the percentage not covered within the contract price by Medicare or any other company on to you. This is where a supplemental plan or a very fat wallet will have to be utilized.

If you have not paid off your deductible for the year, Medicare does not currently do a lump sum attachment to any dollar figure you owe. What that means in simple terms, is that every time you have a balance owed, Medicare will deduct a percentage of your deductible until it is paid off. In dollar amounts, this means that you will pay part of the balance owed (the 20%) and Medicare will pay part. The theory here is that it is easier for the consumer to pay off the deductible in small payments with each bill rather than having no help with each until the deductible is paid.

I want to stress here to contact your Medicare office if you have questions about specifics. Insurance coverage changes. As careful as I have been in creating this book, there is a time lapse between writing and publication. Changes may have occurred. CHECK WITH YOUR CARRIER FOR THE MOST UP TO DATE INFORMATION ON COVERAGE.

I have found the Medicare customer service people to be very helpful and very informative. Their answers have been, for me through the years, clear and concise. If I am holding a bill in my hand, the customer service rep can see it on her computer screen. However, as positive as my experiences have been, I have one thing that is an issue. Hold time. I've discovered in my area that calling on a Monday or Friday means I could probably cook Thanksgiving dinner before someone picks up the call. Tuesday and Thursday mornings seem to be the best times to call. The wait time here is usually only a few minutes.

If you prefer other methods of contacting the office, it can be done, in many areas, in person at the local office. I would call ahead and get some idea of the lighter traffic days and generally a sense of the wait time. Also, there is online capability where waiting won't be an issue. With this many possibilities of contact, it is easy to ask questions and get answers.

It is possible you have heard the term primary insurance. If you have Medicare or Medicaid, there are few cases where neither is deemed the primary insurance. This means that the bill for treatment will not be sent to Medicare or Medicaid first. Neither is responsible for the bulk of the bill and, as stated above, in the case of Medicare that is 80%. This becomes important if you have another insurance that should serve as primary. The medical provider's Patient Financial Rep will be able to determine which insurance to bill as primary for all medical treatment resulting in an automobile accident, workers compensation accident, third-party liability injury, treatment for illness or injuries that occurred during military services or if you are still working full-time. Medicare is very strict about who is to be billed primary in these cases. Medicaid will always be billed last if there is any other insurance besides supplements.

SUPPLEMENTAL PLANS (a.k.a. Medigap Plans) This type of plan is meant to do and be just what it says. It supplements the insurance that your primary, usually this is Medicare. When a supplemental is used it is considered secondary. There are so many supplementals and so many variations in each plan within a plan that discussing all would take a book in itself.

I highly recommend seeing an agent who specializes in medical insurance. Yes, I know that with a computer and a cup of coffee you can find your own policy, thank you very much. But unless you are trained in the field, you won't have the same research capabilities that an agent possesses. There is no charge for this service. The agent makes his commission on the policy he writes. I use an agent and I still check.

My cost did not increase in any way that I could find. In fact, I pay less for my supplemental and get more than friends with the same type of policy.

While I won't recommend any specific plan or policy, I do have one that seems to be often overlooked when someone is shopping for a supplemental. This is PLAN F. This plan has more than one version and is available with more than one company. As with any plan there are good points and bad. The good on PLAN F is that it pays all of the 20% that Medicare doesn't pay and that includes the deductible. What that means to you is that you pay nothing. No co pay. No deductible. The cost for this plan is very competitive, often less than most.

The bad part of PLAN F is that it pays nothing on any charge that Medicare doesn't cover. Depending on your medical problems this may be an issue. Be specific when talking to Medicare, an insurance agent or other insurance. What you leave out of the conversation is probably going to cost you money and you can't change policies at will. There are enrollment dates to be considered. In other words, you could be dealing with inadequate coverage for a year until enrollment opens again to change to another plan or insurance company.

*** As of January 1, 2020, Medigap plans sold to new people with Medicare aren't allowed to cover the Part B deductible. Because of this, Plans C and F are not available to people new to Medicare starting on January 1, 2020. If you already have either of these 2 plans (or the high deductible version of Plan F) or are covered by one of these plans before January 1, 2020, you'll be able to keep your plan. If you were eligible for Medicare before January 1, 2020, but not yet enrolled, you may be able to buy one of these plans. **

REPLACEMENTS (a.k.a. Medicare C or Medicare Advantage Plans) There are many plans available that actually offer benefits that seem to exceed Medicare. In some cases, they do but I would suggest caution here for a number of reasons.

First, this type of policy gives you a card and tells you it is the only card you'll need. No matter how it is worded this is a replacement policy not supplemental. This kind of insurance can have co pays. Medicare does not have a co pay. In other words, you pay a certain dollar figure every time you go to the doctor or the hospital.

Second, this kind of coverage can actually cost more per month than you pay for Medicare. Usually, this increase is supposed to be so you will have better coverage. DO YOU? Find out. Ask your doctor what he charges for an office visit, if you don't already know, then ask what your responsibility would be under Medicare or this policy you are considering. They should know. If not, ask the insurance company. Do the same with the hospital. Pick a procedure that you either know you will need or just one that could happen to anyone, a broken arm or something similar. Tell the person in billing what you are trying to do. Most will take a minute to answer your questions.

Now, you have numbers to compare. If the promises made by the insurance company are valid you will be looking at the dollar amounts to support their claims. If they are not valid, you will have just saved yourself a bunch of headaches and possibly thousands of dollars, not just what the company won't pay, but in the higher premiums you might have paid by believing the promises made to you.

This kind of research is time consuming and something most of us won't want to do. However, the stakes are very high here. And worse if you find out later, say a month into the new insurance year, that your policy doesn't deliver on what you thought was promised, you are stuck until enrollment opens again.

MONEY, MONEY, MONEY. That is bad enough, but it is possible that the covered charges are not as comprehensive as you believed. You could end up needing a procedure that Medicare would have covered, and this 'better insurance' doesn't. DO YOUR RESEARCH. ACTUAL INFORMATION, DOLLAR AND

CENTS INFORMATION, IS A BETTER GAUGE THAN PRETTY WORDS ON A PAGE.

Now that we have explored basic information on insurance and Medicare, the next step is using it effectively. Doctor visits are fairly straightforward. In the case of Medicare, if you are being referred to a specialist, you won't need a referral as you do in many private insurances. Many primary care doctors will even make the appointment for you. If you are an independent person, counting on no one's schedule but your own that can be a time saver. If you are a care giver it may not. Below are some tips on making the doctor visit easier and less problematic.

INFORM THE RECORD KEEPER THAT YOU ARE THE CARE GIVER On your, not necessarily your relative's, first visit to the doctor take the time to inform the record keeper that you are the care giver. Give them your name and phone number. Make sure they do more than just nod when you provide the information.

ASK IF THEY HAVE PAPERWORK FOR YOUR RELATIVE TO SIGN SO THAT YOU MAY GET INFORMATION ON LOVED ONE'S MEDICAL SITUATION. The privacy laws in this country do not permit the physician to answer any questions from you without this documentation. Get a copy for yourself and keep it in a safe place.

I have had to fax a copy of their copy more than once over the years because something didn't get scanned into the system or it was lost in a hard copy office. In more than one case it was a time sensitive question, and few offices move quickly in any information requirement situation.

VERIFY THE NECESSITY FOR MULTIPLE VISITS ESPECIALLY IF A CO-PAY IS INVOLVED. Most of us are accustomed to accepting the doctor's word as law without question. If the physician says you need five visits a week such as in a physical therapy situation, the patient doesn't question the decision even if that patient may be silently stunned at the amount of money that number of treatments will mean in co pays. However, you as the patient have the right and should exercise it in asking if those expensive visits can be either spread out in a more financially acceptable fashion or decreased completely. Doctors, in my experience, have little conception about the costs of their choices for the patient.

Example: During a recent visit to a chiropractor I had with a friend of mine, her doctor did want to see her five times a week. She had a very limited income and a substantial co pay. To do the treatments as prescribed would have had serious effects on her financial health. Since I had worked for a Chiropractor/Physical Therapist for a couple of years, I knew that treatments, in some cases, could be reduced for monetary reasons. My employer was actually a doctor who paid attention to such patient issues. I asked the doctor if this was one of those cases and explained the reason as discreetly as possible. Thankfully, the woman understood and agreed that twice a week would work fine if my friend would do the exercises needed at home. Even twice a week was a strain but at least it was doable financially.

DRUG COVERAGE PLANS If your loved one is not on Medicare; the drug coverage portion is often included in private insurance policies. You may be unaware that with Medicare that part of medical care is separate. Separate drug coverage plans vary greatly in cost and coverage. Also, the coverage is usually based on the specific drugs the patient is using. Changes in drugs means changes in coverage. MAKE SURE THAT YOU KNOW THE RULES IN THIS VERY EXPENSE GAME. A SINGLE BOTTLE OF PILLS CAN BE HUNDREDS OF DOLLARS.

The doctor doesn't know your coverage. He changes drugs for many reasons and not all of them are based solely on their effect on your problem. His reason can be as simple as a company Has come out with a new drug. Most conditions have more than one medication that can produce positive results. ASK THE DOCTOR IF YOUR NEW PRESCRIPTION WILL BE COVERED BY YOUR PLAN.

HIS OFFICE CAN CHECK FOR YOU OR YOU CAN CHECK FOR YOURSELF AND CALL HIM WITH POSSIBLE ALTERNATIVES FOR HIS APPROVAL IF NECESSARY.

Example: My husband had stage four lung cancer. His physician prescribed a drug called Megace. Our drug plan paid for the first prescription but sent a letter advising that the prescription was not on their list of covered drugs. The alternative, the only one at the time, offered was not an adequate substitute, according to his doctor. Thankfully, we were in position to afford the original prescription ($100 a bottle) but what if we had not been. He would have suffered because of inadequate insurance coverage or maybe, in order to purchase the drug, we wouldn't have been able to make a mortgage payment or buy food. This is a very common problem right now.

As you can see insurance is a tricky minefield of questions and problems. In an ideal world, each policy would have clearly defined, easily understood guidelines on each medical condition and treatment options. Each type of drug would have a dollar figure attached for coverage purposes. The patient presents the card. The participating doctor accepts. The treatment is done. A reasonable bill rendered.

NO WAY IN THE UNITED STATES MEDICAL COVERAGE UNIVERSE.

Every company is different. Every plan within that company is different. Every doctor charges differently for every procedure. There are brand drugs and generic drugs. One store charges one price for this drug and the same drug in another store is a lot more or a lot less. Supplements are there to help the patient pay less but sometimes those supplements are disguised as replacements and actually cost more. The doctor has as much trouble understanding insurance as the patient. The people working in the insurance department of the physician's office are often hired without any prior training. The amount of help offered by the doctor's office is only as good as the personnel manning it. The insurance companies are required to provide adequate information when asked but most patients and often doctors too, are not aware enough to ask the right questions or are too intimidated to do so.

Having traversed this minefield both ftom a doctor's office prospective and a patient's and a care giver, I have one rule. ASK QUESTIONS. KEEP ASKING UNTIL YOU UNDERSTAND THE ANSWERS AND HAVE A SOLUTION TO THE PROBLEM YOU ARE FACING. THERE ARE ANSWERS.

Bills can be paid on installments. Insurance companies do answer questions about charges being sent to you by the doctor that you thought should have been paid. Hospitals do treat in emergencies. Read the bills you are sent and the reasons you are receiving them. It is amazing how many errors occur that when chased down prove to be the insurance's responsibility or costs that shouldn't have been billed to you at all. You as the care giver will have to be persistent and relentless. Insurance is time consuming, but time well spent when a bill is paid appropriately.

CHAPTER NINE

INTERACTION WITH HEALTH CARE FACILITIES BEFORE LEAVING

As a care giver you will be going to various medical facilities, doctor's offices, emergency rooms and hospitals. Every one of these places has one thing in common besides the medical aspect. You are going to be sitting, waiting for treatment. In the best of cases, the wait will be less than an hour. But I have found, in the cases of a crisis, the situational waiting is going to be much, much longer. In a crisis such as an emergency room visit every minute seems to last an hour and the mind of the caregiver just can't resist creating fear and worry until laying down beside your loved one feels like a really good idea, especially if you can just go to sleep and then wake up when the crisis is past.

When I, as a care giver, realized that waiting was going to be a fact of my life, I turned to my favorite hobby, reading. I took a book with me. That worked fine in practice until the first ER visit that lasted six hours. I finished the book in two and guess what I did for the next four hours? Worried, Worried, WORRIED and scared myself silly with what ifs that didn't occur. I also had to remind myself that yelling at the health professionals for taking so long was not a good idea.

Also, every time I took myself out to the vending machine, which are always a distance from the emergency area in our hospitals, for a bottle of water, the nurse or doctor would come in to give progress reports. I am firmly convinced each had radar. Try getting an update after the fact. Chances are you will not. Remember, this is emergency room. Patients are in crisis. As important as your loved one is in the scheme of things, repeating an update already given is not as important as caring for someone having a heart attack or bleeding profusely.

An answer came out of a procedure that most women follow when having a baby. They pack a bag in preparation for the anticipated event. I packed a crisis bag for me and my loved one with what I believed I would reasonably need in six hours. In my experience through the last forty plus years this has proven to be the average wait for either emergency room visits with or without admission and in-patient surgical procedures. Outpatient procedures can be shorter but, in my family, not by much. Below is listed the items I included and why. Mine is an example. Personalize to your own taste.

TAKE COPIES OF DNR (do not resuscitate order) IF YOUR LOVED ONE HAS ONE, ALSO COPIES OF HEALTH CARE SURROGATE AND POWER OF ATTORNEY AND COPY OF ALL MEDICATIONS YOUR RELATIVE IS CURRENTLY USING AND WHERE IN THE DAILY DOSSAGE HE OR SHE IS. YOU WILL ALSO NEED THE BOTTLES OF PILLS THEMSELVES. MOST HEALTH CARE PROFESSIONALS PREFER TO READ THE BOTTLES RATHER THAN USE YOUR SPELLING OR AN ORAL LIST. I do not leave the legal documents in the crisis bag. I keep those in my handbag which I make sure doesn't leave my sight. Remember, most of the areas you will be in are public ones.

TAKE ANY MEDICATIONS THAT YOU MAY PERSONALLY NEED. DO NOT TAKE BOTTLES WITH YOU. THERE WILL POSSIBLY BE TIMES YOU ARE OUT OF THE AREA OF YOUR CRISIS BAG. LEAVING PILLS UNATTENDED IN BASICALLY A PUBLIC AREA CAN BE RISKY. REPLACING YOUR MISSING PRESCRIPTION WILL

BE DIFFICULT AND YOU WILL CERTAINLY NEED TO NOTIFY THE HOSPITAL OF ANY ISSUE. DO YOU REALLY WANT THIS KIND OF HEADACHE?

Ear buds are important for items that make noise. The first two are my choices, the crosswords were a friend's suggestion and the laptop my daughter's. She has gotten a lot of work done through the years as she has waited with me while a family member has been treated. Make sure to have power cords and/or chargers for long term usage. Having something portable to pass the time makes the waiting a lot easier. There are only so many magazines any one person can read. Don't forget a bookmark or two and pencils with erasers for the crosswords.

PLASTIC BOTTLES OF WATER, JUICE OR SODA FOR YOURSELF. Vending machines are usually not conveniently placed to the emergency area. If you need something as simple as a bottle of water, you are going to be gone for a few minutes. The good news is that the bathrooms are. If you take a bathroom break, be sure to stop at the desk and let YOUR LOVED ONE'S NURSE know. The health care professionals have radar for nature breaks as well as food ones. Doctors with information almost always appeared when I was on some kind of a break. I couldn't take a bathroom in my crisis bag, but I could take beverages.

SNACKS SUCH AS HEALTH BARS OR SOMETHING YOU CAN EAT WITHIN A WRAPPER. Hospitals often have staph in health care areas. YOU DO NOT WANT BE HANDLING YOUR FOOD WITH YOUR BARE HANDS UNLESS YOU HAVE JUST WASHED THEM AND NOT TOUCHED A SINGLE SURFACE BEFORE YOU EAT. Many people will skip this suggestion thinking eating in a crisis just doesn't matter. It does. You are the health care provider for your loved one. Eating is necessary for a healthy body and, if you take pills yourself or are diabetic, your meals are often critically important.

A SMALL NOTEBOOK AND PEN THAT WORKS Making notes is sometimes necessary. Also, I often make lists of things I need to do on the way home, for myself and the one for whom I am caring. Depending on the issue that has brought you to the care facility and the amount of help you have at home, you may have days ahead of you when leaving your loved one is going to be difficult if not impossible. Depending on the condition of your loved one, you may want to run errands on the way home, especially if one of those errands is to pick up a new prescription.

PERSONAL ITEMS Tissues, feminine products—vending may not be available or if it is not filled, hand sanitizer and wipes. Even if the vending machines are stocked it may not be with the brands you use. Plus, don't forget the change issue. At first, I never seemed to have any when I needed it. Learning my lesson, I put a change purse in my bag with about five dollars in small coins and bills. Since you may end up leaving your bag momentarily with your loved one, it isn't wise to have too much money in the bag.

CELL PHONE

A LIGHTWEIGHT JACKET Hospitals and doctor's offices are cold. Much of the equipment used needs to be in lower temperatures than are comfortable for most of us. Take a jacket or sweater that can be tucked into your crisis bag. The alternatives are being wrapped in a hospital blanket like a mummy or teeth chattering chills. Neither one of these is fashion statement.

FINALLY, THE BAG ITSELF The bag will be on surfaces that may or may not be clean and germ free. Using one of the bags similar to the cloth bags for grocery shopping is an excellent solution. When you return home, it is a simple matter to unload your bag and pop it into the washer. Don't forget to repack when it is finished. I actually use two bags and just transfer the materials from the used bag to the clean one. I have had more than one back to back crisis that has taught me the value of this idea. Don't forget to change your books, DVDs etc. when you change the bag. And definitely check your change purse and restock the money.

Now that you have your bag packed, there are some other basic ideas which will save you time and aggravation. When a person takes on the responsibility of another person in addition to the other daily demands there is stress even if it isn't readily apparent. I prefer to minimize that stress anywhere I can. There is a lot I can't do but these simple things listed below I can.

KEEP TRANSPORT VEHICLE FILLED WITH FUEL. If you are following an emergency vehicle with your loved in it down the road, the last thing you want to be doing is stopping for gas. Throughout my care giving years, my car needed fuel the minute the needle on the gauge touched the half full mark. I can't count how many times this one small trick really mattered.

A PACKED BAG FOR YOUR RELATIVE IN CASE OF HOSPITAL ADMISSION. Toothbrush, toothpaste, denture cleaner and adhesive, favorite soap, shaving cream, razor, emery boards Although most care facilities provide these things, I found my relatives really wanted their own things around them as much as possible. A bar of favorite soap, a brand of toothpaste that is familiar is very important to a relative who is among strangers with a body that is in pain or maybe even facing some terrifying treatment.

Choose a going home outfit, including underwear. I also included underwear for the entire stay. There are situations where doing without this is not necessary. The underwear doesn't take up that much room in the bag. Do check with the nurse or doctor if your loved one is admitted being sure your relative can use the underwear. All of my relatives preferred the dignity of wearing undergarments if at all possible.

Slippers should be included if the patient can get out of bed. Make sure the soles are non-skid. Also socks—I prefer the tube variety because you don't have to worry with the fit. If your relative prefers to walk around in socks be sure to get the kind that have the non-skid bottoms. Hospitals do have these but your relative may end up in his own rather than the hospital's. The last thing you or your relative needs is a fall while in a care facility.

Jewelry is discouraged but occasionally one of my relatives insisted on wearing a watch. I kept an inexpensive one just for this purpose. It usually made it home with us but not always.

Eyeglasses and/or hearing aids are necessary in some cases. Make sure the nurse is aware they are prescription and there is a good chance they will come home with your relative.

A book or two if you have hobby readers like most of my relatives were. Paperbacks are less expensive and can be lost or thrown away without too much of a dent in the wallet. If your relative uses something like Kindle be sure to include a charger. Again, keep in mind that things do get lost in a hospital setting. I tried to pack only what I could afford to replace if something came up missing.

Finally, NO MONEY OR VALUABLES. HEALTH CARE FACILITIES DON'T USUALLY HAVE PROVISIONS FOR EITHER. I have had a couple of admissions where the patient was allowed to purchase small items from gift shop carts that came to the rooms. If this is the case, five dollars is usually a usable amount. Or you can check with the gift shop on site and set up a credit account if that is one of their services.

DOCTORS and DENTIST VISITS

All of the information here is based on my experiences and the most likely situations. Please, keep that in mind as you read. This information is meant as a general outline of what can be expected. Your physician's office may be different. The point here is to make whatever procedure you are dealing with work for you and your loved one.

Early appointments, the first or second of the day, generally are the ones that require the least amount of wait time. When making appointments, you may want to consider your relative's normal wake-up time. For the aging population, early rising is often problematic for a variety of reasons. Preference can be as much of a stumbling block as some physical issue. I have never liked starting the day with a small war trying to get my loved one loaded in the car and to the appointment. It is bad enough when we share the same living arrangement. If it is an off-site living arrangement, it means I have to get up even earlier to get ready then drive to his/her home and get my relative in the car. I'm already tired just thinking about the times I had to do just that.

After the first couple, I considered an alternative. The first or second of the afternoon schedule worked very well. Often, we turned the appointment into an outing that included lunch before the visit.

However, if blood work is to be done this may not always be appropriate. If your relative has lab work that requires a fasting blood sugar, this test is common for diabetics and even for non-diabetics during yearly checks, keep in mind the hardship waiting until afternoon will create. Many times, the doctor's office will consider this aspect but, in my experience, as many times as they did, there were more when it was not considered. SPEAK UP. REMIND THE RECEPTIONIST OF WHAT IS BEING REQUIRED. THE DOCTOR GAVE THE ORDER BUT THAT DOESN'T MEAN THE PERSON SCHEDULING THE APPOINTMENT READ IT ON THE SHEET SHE WAS GIVEN.

Also, if you have a distance to travel, which can often be the case with a specialist, let the office know, especially if this is the first visit. Many offices now cancel appointments automatically if a patient does not show up on time. Get an idea of the time it will take for the trip. Build in an extra half hour just to be safe. Even that won't be a guarantee.

Example: My husband had stage four lung cancer. He was undergoing radiation treatment and it was time for his annual physical. The trip from our house to the doctor's office was forty-one miles. The cell reception was very spotty. He was weak the morning of the visit and took longer than normal to get in the car. I had built in extra time because I knew this had happened before. We had a twenty-minute delay for road construction. No cell reception. We arrived at the office and were told we would have to reschedule. We were six minutes late and the office itself was running over an hour behind seeing patients.

My husband was embarrassed and upset because he felt responsible. The receptionist buzzed the PA who wouldn't even consider making an exception. We did not reschedule. Instead, I stopped at his oncologist office, which was on the way home, and apprised them of the situation. The two doctors involved knew each other. I have no idea what was said but my husband did not have to see that particular doctor again. That part of his health care was handled through his oncologist.

I hope your situation is never this extreme. The point is, know the procedure of your relative's physician so that you can utilize it effectively rather than be victimized by it.

LABORATORY VISITS and DIAGNOSTIC TESTS

Many doctors do their own lab work. Some can even do certain diagnostics. However, that doesn't not mean you, as the patient or caregiver, cannot use a lab more conveniently placed or scheduled. If the lab requirements coincide with your visit, that is convenient but, if you have to come back, consider an alternative that is more suitable for your life. So many of us are intimidated by the medical profession or are just too overwhelmed by the situation into which we have been thrust, that looking for an alternative doesn't even occur to us. I haven't met a situation that didn't have options. Most gave me just that extra few minutes I desperately needed or made it just a little easier to cope. Every one of them was worth the time in searching for the option.

Caregiving isn't just one day, one week, one month or one year. Those extra moments add up quickly.

Also, in the case of diagnostic tests, keep in mind any special needs your relative may have. MRI, for instance, are really no-go areas for many people who are claustrophobic. There are open MRIs and stand up ones as alternatives. However, the more specialized versions may not be as conveniently located as the closed version. Also, often diagnostic tests have dyes involved. Be sure to be aware of any reactions your relative may have had in the past. The test descriptions are usually termed with contrast or without. Contrast is the dye part. I personally have a dye reaction. Any diagnostic test to date, including MRI and CAT scans have been done without contrast, meaning without dyes. It is not as effective as with contrast but so far the testing has been sufficient for my needs at the time. Discuss any and all issues with diagnostic tests with your physician. As always you and your relative have the deciding vote. Use it as necessary with the information provided to you.

EMERGENCY ROOM VISITS and HOSPITAL ADMISSIONS

At this stage of life, most admissions will probably arise from an emergency room trip. First, in this situation, you are at some sort of crisis point. If you have a crisis bag with you and your loved one's case for admission, you will have all you need right then. The documentation carried in the crisis bag will make the admission process considerably easier.

However, neither bag nor case will shorten the time you will spend waiting while your relative is evaluated and/or stabilized and finally taken to the room. The hospitals of today are trying to cut the time in the ER down. You are still locked into the small ER cubicle while tests are run and evaluated and a decision on admission is made. Be patient. More than you can see has to occur for an accurate diagnosis.

Also, many hospitals are so crowded that one patient has to be discharged and the room prepared before another can be taken to a room.

Example: I took my husband to the emergency room where he was diagnosed with a ruptured appendix. He stayed in the emergency room overnight not only waiting for a bed but for the surgical procedure to be performed. It wasn't an ideal situation by any means but none of the hospitals in the area had any room either.

Emergency rooms usually have televisions but be aware of your neighbors with the sound control. Meals are available for both you and your relative (depending on condition). Be sure to check with your relative's health care giver about being fed. Trays for patients are usually not automatically ordered. In the scheme of things in an emergency room setting, feeding patients and/or family members doesn't seem to be a high priority. It is amazing to me how often this is overlooked in an emergency room setting. Be especially aware of this issue if you are care for a diabetic or are one yourself. Do not bring in food from outside or from other areas of the hospital without checking with the health care professional in charge of your loved one.

More often than not emergency rooms are cold enough to refrigerate food. If your relative is prone to chills, make sure you ask the nurse for extra blankets the moment your loved is taken to his cubicle.

Example: My father was especially prone to chills because he had leukemia. The minute he was popped into bed, I asked for blankets and socks as he would stay warmer better with his feet covered. In a couple of extreme cases, I asked if he could have heated blankets. Most hospitals have these and many doctors, in this area anyway, do as well.

It you are taking your family member to the hospital from a doctor's office, most hospital require you enter through the emergency room. I know it seems redundant and from a patient's standpoint it is. However, getting angry about procedure doesn't work well. Be as calm as possible. Remember, your relative is watching you cope. Try not to make it harder on either of you.

I have only one instance where I took one of my relatives directly from a doctor's office to the hospital without the emergency room. I have to say it was the easiest hospital admission I have ever had. The town was small as was hospital. The doctor was well known. He picked up the phone and called the hospital. I drove over. Someone with a wheelchair met me at the car. With a smile and a bit of conversation with my father, he was eased into a wheelchair then through the main door down two halls and into a freshly prepared room. They even had heated blankets waiting that the doctor had ordered because Pop had been chilled in the office. From door to door it was less than twenty minutes. I wish all of my interactions with doctors and hospitals had been this smooth and patient caring.

If you are taking your relative to the hospital for an outpatient or in-patient procedure you will have instructions from the doctor involved and from the hospital itself. Follow them. Every facility and procedure is different. I won't try to outline any routine here. However, don't be afraid to ask questions or ask for slight tweaks if you have some kind of problem with what you are being told to do. Most facilities will try to work with you but none of them can if you don't communicate the problem.

PROBLEMS

No matter how careful everyone is, including you, problems do arise. There are many avenues of resolution available to you. However, most people I have encountered through the years don't seem to realize this. I am going to outline the basics.

Hospital setting when your relative has been admitted Case managers are a good source. Usually there is one per floor for medium to large hospitals. This is the person to see for an overview of your relative's care. You can also get basically the same information from the nurse in charge of your relative's care, but he/she will have a number of patients and limited time. The doctor can also be a source, but the time constraints are multiplied in this case as most will have private practice demands as well.

If the case manager has not addressed your problems to your satisfaction (this has only happened one time for me in all the years this position has existed) you can ask for a patient advocate if the hospital has one or the head of nursing if it doesn't or if it is a nursing issue or if you aren't sure.

If none of those work, there is a hospital administrator's office. You probably won't speak directly to whoever that person is but I have yet to hear of one that doesn't have an assistant. The one time I had to resort to this step, it was as if the entire medical world stopped to listen to the problem I was having getting my dying mother home when her doctor refused to even meet with us to discuss discharge. To this moment, no one, medical or civilian, ever understood the man's behavior. But I got my mother home because that a tiny dynamo, the PA to the administrator, in stilettos wasn't going give up on getting answers and results. Because of her it took about twelve hours to achieve the impossible. My mother died less than 48 hours later in my home instead of hospital she did not want.

Hospital Setting with an Emergency Room Issue A word of caution here. Emergency problems are harder to detect for someone unfamiliar with the medical issues involved. Emergency rooms work on the more critical patients first. No matter how important your loved one is to you, no matter whether you have already been waiting a long time for a doctor to see you or even give you answers, unless your relative is the most critical patient in the ER, you will wait until the critical are dealt with first. Keeping that in mind, occasionally problems do arise.

As a care giver, you know your loved very well. Use that knowledge. Pay attention to what your relative looks like, how they are feeling and talking to you. Color changes, voice changes and chills or fever are caution if not red lights. If you are waiting for care or are in the process where tests are being done with people popping in and out, let the medical professional know what you are seeing. Again, keep in mind that you are not a doctor. This is a very fine line here and can be tricky but the people for whom I cared mattered a great deal to me and they were not dying on my watch. If the medical staff addresses the problem,

Great. If not, you will need to take further action. Calling the doctor involved, if there is one, is one avenue. Going out to the admissions desk and asking to speak to the nursing supervisor is another. A patient advocate if the hospital has one is very useful in this kind of case. I have only had a couple of instances of problems in the ER and all were handled within the ER procedure.

Example: My father was feeling very unwell one afternoon and it was not during office hours for his doctor. We drove him to the emergency room. It was jammed with people when we got there. Minutes waiting turned into an hour. I spoke to the nurse about the length of time and got an adequate explanation and a couple of blankets because my father was getting very chilled. She even came over to check on him as he sat patiently waiting. Another hour went by. Even I could see that the list was still full. No matter how many patients were seen, two would come in even worse. However, my father seemed to be changing before my eyes. His color was not good and he was drooping in the chair as though he was about to slide to the floor. I alerted the nurse. She was definitely busy but promised to check on him as soon as she could.

I have never been an alarmist but some part of me was screaming something was terribly wrong. I called his doctor, got his service and asked for an immediate return call. He called me back and I explained the problem and my concerns. He all but told me I was overreacting but that he was on his way to the hospital for rounds and would stop by the ER to check on Pop. A few minutes later, the nurse came over, checked on my father and a few minutes after that he was taken into one of the exam rooms.

From that moment on things changed dramatically. No one was interested in getting the usual information. My father was going critical with renal failure. The ER doctor and his physician, who did stop by to check, was very busy trying to stabilize Pop. In case you don't know what, renal failure is, it is the kidneys shutting down. Death is usually not far behind.

Pop survived. His doctor came as close as I have ever heard a doctor come to apologizing for not listening. Pop had actually only been in the emergency room about three hours. However, had I not continued to monitor him and approached the desk to report the changes I was seeing, he could have died waiting.

Doctor Setting: This next section addresses a very common problem in the care giving world. Doctors often, when a care giver is present, speak to the care giver rather than the patient. Beware of how the doctor handles the conversational setting on your initial visit. If your relative is very aware and involved in day to day activity, make sure the doctor speaks to your relative not to you. You are the listener here, not the focus. If there is some kind of impairment that reduces your relative's involvement in his care, then having you as the conversational focus can be more effective.

This situation should be addressed before you see the doctor. Introduce yourself to the nurse or assistant who comes to take the vitals. Explain your role and any impairments if any exist. Make sure the information is noted on the records for the doctor's information. Remember, your loved one wants to keep his independence as long as possible. His health and his body are very intimate subjects. No one enjoys being talked over in this kind of situation.

Example 1: When my parents and I visited their doctor together for the first time, a doctor they had had for a number of years, he focused his conversation and maintained eye contact with me throughout the visit. No matter how often I tried to redirect his attention, he kept repeating the same behavior. My mother, a retired RN, was livid. My father was upset because she was upset and on his own account as well. Obviously, the doctor could have handled the situation better. The problem was corrected but it was messy to deal with and the doctor was annoyed because, 'well none of his other patients complained'. Maybe not, but what were they thinking when they were being relegated to just being a body without a mind or feelings?

Example 2: About a year ago I had an opportunity to observe a doctor leading interns or residents through rounds in a large teaching hospital. I watched the man try to talk to my husband who was in the last stages of advanced lung cancer. His cognitive skills had been reduced to almost zero from my point of view and he had difficulty speaking and articulating what he needed or wanted. This doctor talked over him, certainly teaching those gathered around my husband's bed but, in my opinion, not considering what my husband's needs were. After the physician left, two of the students stayed behind to gather more information from my husband. One of them actually noticed that my husband wasn't having much success talking.

They turned to me for answers. In the course of the conversation, I asked a few questions. One of them was about the way some doctors relate to the aging population. By the time both had stopped looking startled and started explaining what was actually being taught, all three of us realized that patient interaction had had little or no place in the educational process.

It had long been my thought but to find, in this educational system anyway, patient relations were not taught is something I think should be addressed. We are not just bodies but minds. As a care giver, remembering that yourself and reminding those caring for your loved one is important.

Most people tend to bow to the doctor in all things without question. Modern medicine is a long way from that family physician you have had since you took your first breath. There is a lot of good in the technology but there is bad as well. Equally, the doctor's office itself is much bigger in many cases and the doctor is farther from the actual workings of his workplace. Many have office managers.

Depending on the problem an office manager is a very good addition. Scheduling issues, billing and overall response to such problems as call backs and messages left, in over words, non-medical problems, the manager can affect resolutions. If it is a billing problem, you will want to start in the billing department, assuming there is one. If not, start with the office manager. Get names of everyone with whom you deal, first, for referencing if you end up speaking to more than one person. Secondly, connecting with anyone by using that person's name usually results in a much better contact than one where you appear to not care enough to even remember with whom you are dealing.

If you are having a medical problem, such as a doctor spending three minutes barely listening to you and never making eye contact, consider getting a new doctor. Most areas have more than one doctor for any specialty. You need not suffer a doctor that barely acknowledges you exist or a doctor who does not take your concerns seriously or a doctor who requires weekly visits without adequate explanations. Or, this my favorite, a doctor who has multiple PAs for you to see but never even sticks his nose in your cubicle for months or even years at a time. I have had doctors like this but not for long.

If you are on Medicare there is actually a requirement for physically seeing a doctor per year. Medicare is not talking about a PA in this case. Because insurance and its requirements change so often and currently Medicare is changing a great deal, I strongly suggest, if you are in an office with the PA system of medical care, if you have never or rarely seen the doctor you pay for, call Medicare and find out what the current requirement is. If your doctor is not meeting it, let Medicare know.

Finally, being abrupt with health care providers is not smart. You gain nothing for your relative and the health care worker is just as human as you are. Most are going to do their job to the best of their ability but what about that one or two who lets you and your relative wait for an extra hour just because you lost your temper?

If you encounter a problem, address it calmly and clearly. Be kind. Most people respond more favorably to kindness than temper tantrums. This is especially a better course of action if you are going to be dealing with the facility or persons in the future. It is amazing how long the memory can be for a person who has screamed at you, no matter how justified it might be.

CHAPTER TEN

IN HOME CARE AFTER HOSPITALIZATION

Your loved one has been in the hospital and is now going to be discharged into your care. With so much paperwork and so many patients, you may encounter a hospital that discharges around the clock. Even though the ones I have encountered that say this, the truth is that the actual discharge takes place mostly in daylight or early evening hours. However, hospitals do discharge on weekends as well. This after normal business hours can be problematic for the caregiver for a number of reasons.

Medications I have yet to have a patient discharged to my care who came to me without a handful of prescriptions. There are certain discount stores that offer extended pharmacy hours but not all locations follow this schedule. Nor do all pharmacies. Know your pharmacy hours of operation. The doctor may not even tell you that he is making out new prescriptions or changing dosages on old ones. ASK. DO NOT LET THE DOCTOR WALK OUT OF THE ROOM WITHOUT FINDING OUT THE DETAILS OF MEDICATIONS. THE HOSPITAL CAN'T PROVIDE MEDICATIONS FOR YOU TO TAKE HOME SO THAT YOU CAN HAVE TIME TO FILL PRECRIPTIONS. THINK LIABILITY.

If your relative is being discharged with prescriptions and there is a conflict in getting them filled, tell the doctor. He can arrange to either have part of the dosage administered before your relative is discharged or possibly even arrange a better time for discharge. Also, in some cases, you may use the discharge procedure time, it often takes as much as six hours to get the job done, to slip out and get the prescriptions filled. This is out of procedure but definitely to the patient's advantage in that he or she will go home with the proper meds and not skipping dosages while you wait for a pharmacy to open.

Example: I was visiting a friend in the hospital. Her stepdaughter was my friend and her care giver. The doctor came in to see her and decided that she was doing so well that he would set the discharge in motion. It was Sunday morning. My friend and her stepmother used a pharmacy close to their homes which did not have Sunday hours. Neither thought to ask the doctor about the prescriptions he was writing. He was just about to walk out of the room when I did ask and explained the problem. He arranged to discharge so that my friend's medications could be given prior to leaving the hospital so that my friend would be able to have the prescriptions filled the following day. As it happened the discount store close by did have most of them and the part of the list was filled while we waited through the discharge process.

Medical Equipment Like the prescriptions, you may have discharge instructions that include some sort of medical equipment, bedside commode, walker, cane, oxygen tanks and supplies, hospital bed with rails, etc. Insurance coverage for this kind of thing varies greatly and the hospital staff will not have checked, nor will the doctor be writing the order.

Don't assume because it is in the discharge paperwork, that you won't be getting out your wallet. If you are doing an after-hours discharge, use a phone to find out if you can get whatever equipment you will need. Even trying to handle a patient who simply needs assistance walking from bed to bathroom becomes a nightmare if you have never done it before or if you a smaller person trying to help a much larger relative. If you do not have the proper equipment, don't be intimidated about saying so.

Remember: Your loved one becomes your responsibility the moment you leave the hospital. If you are going home with a patient who is bed ridden and tends to roll around when sleeping, a bed with rails is a necessity not a luxury. Discount stores and pharmacies don't have floor models of these items. There is at least a full day of ordering and scheduling before you will see a bed with rails to protect your relative from going crashing to the floor. The same can apply to oxygen equipment depending on what is required.

If there is conflict, sometimes they do arise, explain the situation. If the staff is not adapting to your needs, contact the doctor if possible or the case manager for help. If that doesn't work, contact the supervisor of nursing. After hours discharging makes solving problems difficult as most hospitals don't have the full staffing in the supervisory offices. Most run on normal business hours schedules. If you have been advised that discharge may take place on a weekend or after six, talk to the nurse or doctor about what, if any special equipment will be needed to make your loved one's transfer to your home or theirs safe for them and workable for you.

Transporting your loved one home This is something that many overlook. If you are bringing home a loved you can walk but you have a flight of stairs to climb to get to the front door, can he or she make it? Find out before you leave the hospital. The care giving staff is not filled with mind readers. Let the doctor, nurse and physical therapist, if there is one, know about any issues that any exist.

Examples:

Stairs—Your relative may have been up and down these many times but a hospital stay can reduce mobility, strength or endurance. What was possible before the stay may not be now.

The transport vehicle—Your loved one may be accustomed to the vehicle you normally use but will it work now? Is it easy to slip into or most your relative lift his or her legs over a floor ledge just to get in the car? If there has been a surgical procedure involved, the strain of lifting his or legs may not be possible or even desirable.

Parking and unloading—Is there a long distance from where you need to leave the vehicle and where you enter the home? Is your loved one capable of moving that far?

Placement in the home—Where is the bedroom for your relative? Again, are there stairs?

As you can see, there is more to taking your relative home than just popping them into your vehicle. If you have complications, let the doctor and staff know. Depending on the situation, a non-emergency transport may be necessary. The hospital should check to verify that your insurance will cover the cost. Regardless of the answer, use the phone and verify for yourself. Your relative is the bill to party and it is yours or his/her responsibility to make sure of coverage. Non-emergency is not cheap.

In home care You will be advised that your loved one is eligible for in home care during the discharge procedure. Most discharges I have handled or been involved with will offer a choice in companies to provide that care. If you are a first timer, this can be a problem. How do you choose the right one? Hospitals do not recommend one company above another. The hospital usually will provide brochures on the companies. Take a moment to read what you are given. In the beginning, I kept the brochures so I could change companies if I wasn't satisfied with the care being given to my relative. I have been fortunate not to need to make any changes. But, since that first time, I researched the home care givers in each area when I moved with my relatives. That first time or having to choose with only promotional material as a guide was not something I wanted to repeat.

In home care, comes in a number of forms: physical therapy, occupational therapy, speech therapy, nursing (wound care etc.) and hygiene. Currently, Medicare has guidelines that begin at the time of discharge and restart with each hospitalization. The guidelines and the number of days allowed are clearly stated. The hospital should be able to indicate how much help you can expect. However, mistakes can be made with the best of intentions.

Contact Medicare directly to confirm the information you have been given or to simply find out if you haven't been told anything. Also, keep in mind insurance is constantly changing. Make sure you have the most current information. Having help, when you bring your loved one home, means you can be assured of having a trained professional overseeing your relative's care in the recovery process. In today's hospital care system, patients are sent home as soon as possible. Every doctor any of my relatives had made the same comment when discharging: "You will heal better at home than here."

Most of the time, your relative will be eligible for more than one professional. This can work to the care giver's advantage in more ways than just the obvious.

Example: My father had open heart surgery. When he was discharged, he needed wound care for the harvest site in his thigh for the bypass, physical therapy to regain his strength safely and occupational therapy for the various new ways he needed to do things until he was healed. In short, I would be hosting three different health care givers in my home. Those care giving professionals would be checking his vitals and tracking his progress. Most visits lasted an hour to ninety minutes and each professional only came once or twice a week. Rather than have all of them coming on the same day, I chose to stagger the visits so that my father had someone checking him every day for the length of time Medicare allowed.

This practice not only meant that a professional was looking at him and monitoring the slightest changes in his condition but it meant that during his treatment times, I could run to the pharmacy or the grocery store for those small errands that seem to pop up the minute you need to stay at home around the clock. None of the care givers needed me to be present for his treatment so those hours allowed me to take care of issues I would not have been able to otherwise or, at least, not as easily.

Another advantage, and in many ways the most important advantage, is the expert eye of the skilled health care professional. In my father's case, despite our best efforts, his wound was not healing as it should. Because I had staggered the care givers, it was actually the physical therapist who noticed the change in the site. She brought it to my attention and contacted my father's nurse. In less than an hour a nurse arrived to assess the change. The wound had become infected. The doctor was called, and medications were prescribed. Before the day was over, my father's situation was being handled. He made a great recovery from that point on. However, had he not had his care staggered that way, his nurse would not have seen the site for another day and the infection would have progressed further and would have been harder to control. Now, let's talk about the roles of the professional care givers.

Nurses are assigned to not only care for the patient in the home in this recovery phase but to make assessments both of the patient and the home environment. It is their job to help you understand what you need to do for your relative and what you can do in the home to make that job easier. They are also there to check your relative's physical and emotional condition and to do any wound care needed. It is your responsibility to let the health care professional know if you have any concerns.

They cannot address problems if you don't tell them they exist. Make a list of questions and concerns. USE IT. WRITE DOWN THE ANSWERS. DON'T DEPEND ON YOUR MEMORY ESPECIALLY IF MEDICATIONS ARE INVOLVED. READ YOUR INFORMATION BACK TO THE PROFESSIONAL IN CASE YOU HAVE MISUNDERSTOOD. And, this is very important, pay attention to your relative's state of mind. Fear, frustration, anxiety and despondency are very possible in the healing phase. If you notice any mood changes that surprise or worry you bring it to the attention of the nurse. Don't be embarrassed about this last step. You are in a crisis situation and you are probably not a trained health care giver. Mistakes are very easy to make here. I would much rather make them on paper or verbally than on someone I love.

Also, your nurse will advise you if supplies are being shipped to you for your relative's care. Most of my supplies have been of the wound care variety, protective gloves, dressing materials, disinfecting solutions etc. I create a special table for all these items so that when the nurse or I need them, they are readily available. Also, a closed top trash container should be near the bed for discarded items. I would highly recommend NOT putting the trash can near the clean and, in some cases, sterile supplies. The cleaner this area is kept the safer it is for your relative. Staph doesn't just exist in hospitals. Pay attention to the amount of materials and any shortages. The nurse will take care of reordering.

Physical therapists are assigned to help your relative recover mobility and strength. The term 'range of motion' will be a part of your life. Your therapist will give you a definition and explain the exercises that you will oversee when the therapist is not present. It is essential for patient's best recovery that you follow the instructions carefully and do the exercises as often as needed. If you do not understand, ASK QUESTIONS.

Example: The first time I faced this situation was with my father's open-heart surgery. I knew what range of motion was, but I didn't know all the details about the exercises. I felt like a kid trying to understand an adult. I even apologized for asking the PT to repeat the instructions. She put me at ease with a very simple statement. "I would rather have to repeat instructions so that you can understand than to leave here not realizing I am leaving my patient with someone who can't support him until I come again." Unfortunately, in today's health care environment, the relative of a patient is often in the position of working in lieu of a trained professional. It's a daunting and scary concept but it is also an inescapable one.

Physical therapists also decide what, if any, mobility aids the patient needs in the present and in the future. It is the therapist who decides a walker or cane is necessary and the therapist who helps make sure the one obtained is adjusted properly for your relative. It is also a therapist who ultimately decides with the doctor if a wheelchair will be necessary. If the condition warrants, a special assessment is made to determine if the patient qualifies for a manual or electric wheelchair. Manual is currently the only wheelchair covered by Medicare unless some impairment in the hands or arms exist to make using a manual chair difficult if not impossible. Only then will Medicare cover the cost. In other words, a patient with Medicare who needs a wheelchair can't just request an electric one. The patient must qualify.

Also, Medicare does not currently cover any part of the cost for a wheelchair lift so that the chair can be taken in a vehicle to another location. Lifts are not cheap and do not fit all vehicles. Some insurance won't cover these costs either if Medicare doesn't cover any of the charges. You will need to check carefully with your insurance, Medicare and any supplement. If your relative is a veteran, it is possible the lift will be covered through the VA. Also, if the veteran qualifies, his or her chair could be covered by the VA as well. Checking benefits of all sources is essential in a wheelchair situation.

Wheelchairs are designed to give a patient mobility but the lack of funding through Medicare severely limits that mobility to the home environment when the lift is not covered. This is one place, in my opinion, where the qualification standards need to be revisited.

Occupational therapists are assigned when a patient needs training in how to cope with everyday tasks, chores such as putting on socks or shoes when one has difficulty in bending over, picking up items, even taking a shower when mobility has been impaired. Some of these situations are simply temporary and some permanent. The occupational therapist is there to teach your relative how to cope and you how to relate to this new change in circumstances. There may be exercises here as well. At the very least, practice will be involved. The mobility saving devices are simple to use, things such as the grabber that can pick up paper from the floor and the extra-long shoehorn that makes leaning over to put on shoes unnecessary.

However, rarely are the first attempts of use the best attempts. I have found that trying the devices for myself, even with unimpaired mobility, helps me to understand the problems of using the devices at all. No device, no matter how clever the design, replaces the real ease that once existed with muscles and limbs. Your loved is very apt to be frustrated by the simplest aid. If you have tried the device yourself, you will be better able to understand his/her reaction.

Example: My father, after his open-heart surgery, had been told to avoid leaning over and picking up things, even things as light as a sheet of paper. No one wanted the staples closing the incision to shift and part. His occupational therapist had given him a grabber. This one was even better than the one he had been using for years when his knees just wouldn't bend to reach for something. This grabber had two pieces of vinyl coated metal and a really nice spring load trigger that could lock the device onto the object being collected. He used it for everything.

The problem he had was a simple one. He kept leaving the thing in different areas of his suite and would, invariably, sit down in his favorite chair and discover the grabber was in the kitchen where he had last used it. It only took two days for me to contact the pharmacy and purchase a second grabber for his chair. The cost was surprisingly inexpensive and worth it to me to give him the freedom of his own home. However, within two more days, I now had two grabbers across the room from where he sat. Since, neither he nor I wanted to be tripping over dozens of the things, we decided to tie the grabber to the chair using a cord that was long enough for him to use the device but not long enough to trip him up when he left the chair. We had a good laugh over our solution for the migrating grabber. It worked too.

Home help aides I have run into many different names for these very helpful people. I have seen CNA, hygiene staff person etc. Generally, in the companies with which I have worked, these individuals are assigned when help is needed for tasks such as bathing and moving large patients around in an extremely limited mobility situation. A home help aide does not generally come every day. In situations such as turning your loved one in bed to prevent pressure point sores, the solution would be multiple rotations per day. Clearly, a single visit would not address this problem. However, there are devices that can be connected to special bed pads to reduce the risk of bed sores.

Example: We had an aide assigned to help us with my mother, a very large woman well over 275 pounds with severe osteoporosis and arthritis. Any movement at all hurt her unbearably. With the help of pain pills, an aide and my father, we were able to keep her clean and fresh with as little pain as possible. While she was getting her shower, I was able to change her linen and pillows. The process was not a short one and it wore all of us out but within an hour, she was again in bed, hair brushed and the makeup she insisted on having applied.

As you can see, there is help available and most of these options, in my experience, are discussed with you and your loved one at the time of discharge or, in some cases, during a doctor's visit when the situation has changed for your relative. However, there have been occasions when no one thinks to outline for you, the care giver, the help available to you. With this demanding, twenty-four/seven job, you do need help.

Check with Medicare, your loved one's insurance, both primary and secondary or supplemental. Each will answer your questions and give you the options available for your situation. If the options don't cover your needs, contact your local church or senior center. Often either or both will have some aid to offer.

Remember, the more help you accept the better care you can provide. Even with the help of family, you are still one person handling a mentally, emotionally and physically demanding task. Accepting help doesn't make you weak. It makes you smart and, most of all, helps you stay strong for the ones you love.

Problems with home care do arise. Some are simple, such as scheduling. When I have my first contact with the home health care company, usually by phone, I make it clear in a nice way, that appointments for care need to be as accurate as possible. In other words, if the nurse is supposed to arrive at 9am, 4pm won't do. Be polite but be firm. Remember, this is a paid service and you are the one writing the check whether it is to the insurance that pays the bill or to the company directly. To date, all of my in-home care appointments have stayed within an hour range of arrival with no phone call for an explanation. In other words, 9am can show up as early as 8am or as late as 10am.

If the delay exceeds this, the office or the health care professional needs to use the phone to let me know the new arrival time. I have occasionally run into resistance on this procedure, but it isn't difficult to circumvent. There are other companies that offer the same service. A timely reminder often does the trick. And, you as the care giver have the final say. If the scheduling does become an issue, if the company does not co-operate, contact the insurance that pays the bills. There are remedies and the insurance people know them, in my experience.

Equally, if you should be unfortunate enough to run into that one healthcare professional who only gives lip service to his job description, address your concerns directly to the company. Home health care exists to aid you in caring for your relative, not to just stand around pretending to do a good job. If the company does not address the issue, in other words send a different person, contact the insurance company with your problem and the fact the company has not addressed the issue. A contract exists between the insurance and the health care company. Terms are clearly stated. There are certain standards of care required. Insurance takes this kind of problem seriously, but it can't fix what it doesn't know. It is up to you to make the call.

CHAPTER ELEVEN

MEDICAL EQUIPMENT

Medical Equipment is a big term covering a lot of ground. Since I am not an expert, I am talking about this subject from the prospective of a care giver. That means for you the reader, simple terms and simple uses. And sources both for the equipment itself and for the professional when needed. Also, as far as private insurance is concerned, the coverage is very specific and, in all the cases I know, must be ordered by the doctor to even be considered eligible. If time permits, check with your insurance company about the qualifications you will need to meet. The equipment isn't cheap and usually more than one thing is needed. Where Medicare is concerned, my experience has been that the qualifications required haven't been as difficult to meet as those my earlier care giving had encountered. Again, every case is different and what worked for me may not work for you. Checking with your loved one's carrier is the best answer.

The first category of medical equipment is that collection of products and devices that you may need when your patient comes home from a care facility. If the patient is bed ridden, obviously you will need a bed. No, your personal furniture will not do. The average bed is too low for you to handle the tasks that your loved one will need. Even abs of steel will weep at bending over the bed fifty or sixty times a day plus all the other tasks you will be tackling. A double, queen or king bed will make the situation even worse. When you add to the fact, your relative may try to turn that one time when you aren't looking and fall out of bed because there are no rails, you should be able to see why a hospital bed is a necessity.

A hospital bed raises and lowers very easily. It has rails to keep your relative safe from falling. The head and the foot can be raised or lowered to give your loved one different position for eating, reading, watching television. It also has lockable wheels so that it can be pushed around the area if necessary. And it has a waterproof mattress which can be very important in keeping your loved one dry and fresh.

Also, if your loved one is especially tall, be sure to remind the person who is ordering the bed for you. Hospital beds do come in extended lengths and in special widths if your loved one is larger than average. You will need special fitted linen as well which should come with the bed.

Bed table. I'm sure you have seen these in the hospital. Yes, I know you have tables. Put a hospital bed beside them and you will discover they are too low and don't stretch across your loved one's lap for meals. Clean up a few spills and change and wash the linen a few dozen times and you'll see this adjustable table has more uses than you thought.

Pressure mattress This one was new to me with the last relative for whom I cared. My relative had a staph infected bed sore he got in the hospital. It was critical that he be turned on a regular basis, hourly not daily. He was a big man and turning him for a woman a hundred pounds lighter and a foot shorter and over sixty to boot was not a great solution. The doctor ordered a pressure mattress just like the one he had in the hospital. The mattress looked something like an egg carton and attached to a small motor you could barely hear when it was activated. The mattress pulsed beneath my loved one's body length, keeping the pressure points constantly changing. The device was very comfortable according to my relative and especially because he didn't have to go through the pain of being turned every hour.

Wedges These are foam type product is triangular in shape and come in sizes. They are primarily used on a regular bed (one that can't raise head or foot).

Oxygen equipment This equipment is highly specialized and requires some training for in home use. I won't try to outline the details here because I am not a trained professional. I will say that I have had three of my relatives come home with oxygen equipment of all sizes and types. Each also came with extra tubing and bottles for emergency supplies. All had training for me until I was completely comfortable with what I had to do with each of my loved one.

Write down any instructions given by the professional and keep them with the manuals that may accompany the equipment. I tape a clear, zippered bag to the equipment with my handwritten notes inside. If I question anything I am doing, I CHECK MY NOTES. You should also have been given a contact number for any problems with the equipment. USE IT IF ANYTHING LOOKS UNUSUAL. BETTER TO QUESTION AND BE TOLD THAT EVERYTHING IS FINE THAN TO DISCOVER YOUR LOVED ONE IN DISTRESS BECAUSE OF EQUIPMENT FAILURE OR YOUR MISTAKE.

Bedside commode Unless you are a plumber, toilets aren't a favored topic of conversation. However, if your loved one comes home with mobility restrictions, you will find you are a big fan of the bedside commode. This aide comes in sizes to fit the need of the user. The legs are adjustable for comfort and patient ease. There are heavy duty versions for those who are larger than normal. The adjustments are easy to make but, if possible, let a professional do it for you. One click more or less sometimes makes a big difference in safety as well as comfort and ease of use.

Chairs I am not referring to wheelchairs here. These are chairs that resemble a lounger. These are helpful for the patient who has limited mobility but doesn't quite qualify for a wheelchair or who is in some special recovery situation. Primarily, these chairs allow the patient to sit in comfort, change position for himself without overtaxing limited strength and to have feet and legs elevated. The ones I have seen are moisture proof and can be used with the bed table if necessary.

MOBILITY AIDS

Canes no longer come only in black or gray pipe. They come in colors or patterns with curved handles or straight. Lightweight, foldable and some that stand on a tiny tripod base so that it can stand alone are a few of the design possibilities. Many have loops on or near the handle so that the user can retain possession of the cane if his/her hand slips off the handle or top. The important issue here is don't just pick up a cane and hand it to your loved one.

Canes must be adjusted to the height of the user for maximum benefit. Too short and the user throws his/her balance off by leaning forward. Too tall and the user has no way to really use the cane for balance. Both situations greatly increase the risk of falling. Get a professional to adjust the cane height.

Walkers are for those who need more support than a cane can provide. Again, the walker comes in sizes for those who need a device to be wider or to bear more weight. Also, for convenience there are foldable walkers that make taking it in a car very easy. You have probably seen walkers with tennis balls on the front two legs. This makeshift arrangement allows the user to slide the walker rather than pick it up with each step. While the tennis balls do work, they can get wet or dirty. I prefer the Teflon slides that are available. They are very inexpensive and are barely noticeable on the ends of the front legs. Also, for those who need or want to carry items when using the walker, there are baskets that hang on the front. There are a couple of sizes and shapes available as well.

Example: My mother used a walker, but she didn't like her purse laying in the basket. I attached a Velcro strap to the front bar and hung her purse from there. It left the basket free for items when she shopped and kept her purse in, what she considered, a safer place.

Rollater Walkers come in three wheel and four-wheel designs. There is also a heavy-duty design as well. A rollator walker differs from a walker in that each leg has a wheel. This creates an ease of forward motion. The wheels all have locking mechanisms similar to the brakes on a bicycle. Most have various basket options.

Three Wheel Rollator Walker weighs 12 to 16.5 pounds. The wheels will also vary in diameter. All the models with which I am familiar fold for easy transport and storage. Also, all have weight maximums. When ordering or choosing one of these, I would again suggest a professional. Remember this device will not only aid in mobility but balance. Your loved one will be using it in a weight bearing manner. If the equipment is too light, an accident could result.

Four Wheel Rollator Walker weighs approximately 12 to 18 pounds. Like the three legged, the four folds for easy transport and storage. Also, the wheel diameter will vary according to model as will the weight bearing capability. The four-wheel also comes with a seat in some models. This is my personal favorite type of walker. Your loved one has some sort of mobility issue or he/she would not need a walker. This walker, when equipped with a seat, gives your relative the ability to simply sit down when he/she needs to rest. It also means that your loved one can sit down if he/she suddenly feels dizzy which can be a side effect of many medications, blood pressure medicines being just one of many. The first time I had to brace one of my relatives while looking desperately around for a place to seat him was also the last time. I contacted the doctor to ask about a rollator walker. Not all insurances will cover these and if they do there will be qualifications.

Wheelchairs come in a variety of shapes, sizes and weights. There are manual wheelchairs, these are the ones either pushed by another person or propelled by the user. The chairs of this type come in different weights, standard, light and ultralight.

Transport wheelchairs are most often used in care facilities and when your loved one only needs temporary mobility assistance in a home situation. Transport chairs also fold for storage or tucking into a car's back seat or trunk. These are also good in-home settings because the transport chair is narrower than a standard wheelchair. This means that maneuvering in narrow halls or through doors not 36" wide is possible without retro fitting your home. Another advantage, in some cases, is the ability to remove the footrests from the chair. Having a chair where the patient can use his feet to move from place to place can give recovering muscles an easy way to get gentle exercise. This is not something that should be tried without the advice and approval of your physician.

In my experience, these chairs take a bit of effort on the part of the care giver, especially if your loved one is larger than average or if the care giver is shorter. Example: I'm not very tall. When I pushed my overweight mother in her wheelchair, I wasn't high enough to see her feet. I had to be extra careful turning corners and so forth to avoid hitting them.

Standard weight wheelchair starts at 35 pounds and can be self-propelled. Because of the weight of the chair, this is usually not used for long periods a day. In short, moving the chair plus the occupant's weight around for hours is tiring. This type can have fixed leg rests and arm rests or elevating leg rests and removable arm rests. Some models also have an option to raise or lower the height from the floor. This is especially important if the patient has long legs. Having one's knees tucked up almost to the chin is not a comfortable position.

Also, if your loved one is in the chair for an hour or more at a time, consider a foam cushion for additional comfort. While the seats in most I have tried are not uncomfortable I would not call any of them plush. I found my relatives preferred the addition of a cushion. There a number of types available at many pharmacies. I tried each out until I found the one that suited each relative. The prices were not high and in some cases the doctor can write a prescription for the cushion and the insurance will pay. You will need to check with your insurance to be sure.

Lightweight Wheelchairs usually fall in the 28-34-pound range. Because of the lighter weight, this chair can be used with greater ease for longer periods of time. Colors for the frame and upholstery are available as well as other options in leg rests, arm rests and seating sizes and heights. Customization is also possible here depending on the company.

Ultralight Weight Wheelchairs weigh in as low as 14 pounds. Performance and ease of use are the keys in this type of chair. Depending on the company there are many options and configurations from which to choose.

Tilt/Recline Wheelchairs are for those patients who need a reclining back position. This type of chair is usually for those who spend most of the day in a wheelchair and cannot position themselves with ease or at all. The reclining position flexibility helps by relieving pressure problems created from a single, mostly fixed positioning of the body. This type of chair is heavier because of the additional option and therefore not as easy to transport.

Heavy Duty Wheelchairs are built for those individuals needing a large, sturdier design. The weight bearing capability ranges from 300 to 850 pounds. Most options are available on these models. Researching the companies which offer these will give more specific data.

Electric wheelchairs are for those who cannot handle the manual wheelchair. Most insurances do not cover an electric chair simply because the occupant prefers that type. Certain qualifications, especially in Medicare, apply. The person must have some loss of range of motion in the arms or hands or some other specified impairment that would make propelling the chair manually difficult if not impossible. Upgrading at the insured's expense from the qualified chair type may be possible with some insurances. Be sure to check out the possibility if that is your loved one's preference.

Wheelchair lifts or ramps are often necessary for transporting electric wheelchairs. Electric wheelchairs are not easily transported because of weight and bulk. You will need a lift that can be attached to the outside of most cars or trucks or you can, if you have a van and certain types of SUVs, have a lift that mounts inside your vehicle. Usually the lift is operated by a remote device to remove the ramp from the vehicle and lower to the ground where the occupant can just drive on. The occupant then gets off, the chair is strapped down, and the lift is raised with the chair and eased into the vehicle. Lifts come in a variety of styles and uses. There are also lifts that carry chair and occupant into the vehicle. There are also ramps available for loading the electric wheelchair.

Research on the internet will give you an idea of what is available. Before you approach a doctor about the lift, have an idea about what would work best for you and your loved in your situation. Doctors don't always know individual needs the way you do.

However, the insurance industry is not especially helpful with the costs involved in lifts, especially Medicare. At this writing and from previous experience, a lift is not covered at all. I have had various explanations for this denial. To give a person the ability to move with greater freedom in his or her environment and then refuse to at least partially cover the cost of the lift which allows mobility outside the home environment seems counterproductive to me. Should your loved one be a veteran, you should be able to get help with the cost of the lift. Although usually not as expensive as the electric wheelchair, the lift is not cheap. Financial help for this level of freedom is a must for most of us. If insurance, Medicare and the VA can't help, your local Elder Care organization may be able to point you in the direction of private assistance possibilities. There is an Elder Care Locator on the internet for the office closest to you. I have found them invaluable for so many questions when I run into an obstacle.

There is often a problem discussing with your aging loved one the need for assistance. The doctor can write all the prescriptions he wants and even tell his patient that walking unaided is no longer desirable or safe. Your relative will likely even nod in all the appropriate places. You'll breathe a sigh of relief and think you are home free. There is a good chance you are going to discover you have been living in la la land. Mom may not even consider walking with an ugly black cane. Dad may dig in his heels and get a strangle hold on his mule genes and refuse to look at a walker.

"I can walk fine. I am not using that damn cage like an old woman."

"What do mean I need a wheelchair? I just walk slower. You try hopping around at my age and see if you can do it. If I am this much trouble just put me in a home."

Mobility aids seem to have no positive image at all, especially not with the aging population. All of my relatives, even the medically trained ones, dug in their heels and pitched all kinds of temper tantrums about canes, walkers and wheelchairs. And that was when any of them would even discuss the issues.

Sitting down to discuss this issue is often even more frustrating. Reasoning seems to take a backseat, in most cases, to appearances. Mom or Dad doesn't want to look old or frail. He or she has lost the full use of his or her own body and now he or she is pushing around an advertisement of that fact or worse, riding in one.

CHAPTER TWELVE

CHANGING CARE GIVING LOCATION

This chapter is for those of you who have cared for your loved one in one setting and now, because of medical, physical, emotional or financial reasons have to change the location where you will be doing care giving. Or, in the more extreme cases, turn the caring for your loved one over to strangers. This can also be a multistage process with more than one change of location, each placement representing clearly that your loved one won't be with you much longer.

Changing the location is very difficult for both sides.

Realizing you are coming to the end of caring for your loved one is the hardest part of the process of care giving. You have spent months; years being deeply involved in your relative's life. You have cried with them, even if no one but you saw or felt the tears, you have laughed with them and you have loved them. The visits to the doctor are increasing. The emergency room is more a fact of your life and theirs.

Moving from a home environment to an assisted living or extended care facility. So far you and your family, if you have one, have been able to handle your loved one's needs in your home or theirs. This process, no matter how short or long, has reached the end of feasibility. Reasons for changing are as varied as the current living arrangements themselves. Unfortunately, in my experience, the more care and love that the care giver poured into the choice he/she has made to support their loved one through this stage of life often makes it all the difficult when the time comes to change the care giving location.

The care giver can feel deeply that they have failed the loved one, not been there enough, not spent enough time, missed something. If only he/she will work a little harder, do more, be more, the clock will stop and the loved one won't need different than the care giver can give. Most try all these steps and find it just isn't enough. Failure is a bitter taste that's doesn't leave the mind and heart. If only is the beginning so many thoughts and most, if not all, hurt. If I could give a single gift to all the care givers of the world, it would be peace in this stage. Here's why.

You have done everything you believed you could in the days, months and years of your care giving. You were not perfect, no one is, but YOU WERE AND ARE THERE TO THE BEST OF YOUR ABILITY. YOU DID AND ARE DOING WHAT MOST, POSSIBLY EVEN THOSE IN YOUR OWN FAMILY, WOULD NOT DO.

Your loved one, no matter how cantankerous or delightful, knows you have been there. The cranky ones may not show his or her appreciation in obvious ways, but it is there. Example: If you have been reading this book, you know my mother was not in the delightful category. She was in the hospital and it was clear that the nurses and doctors were only maintaining her level of health. I tried to consult with her physician, but he evaded any attempt for a family discussion.

Finally, on a morning when I had just arrived to visit my mother and I could hear her shouting for a nurse when I could see one was just leaving her room, when I could hear patients' complaining about her behavior, I approached the nurses' station and explained my problem. They, too, had given messages to the doctor from us.

The hospital needed relief and so did we. It took twelve hours, a hospital administrator, a case manager who stayed overtime, a hospice liaison and countless hospice people delivering equipment to my house for my mother's care and a medical transport team and my brother riding shotgun to get my mother home.

The first thing she said to me, the only thing she said to me before she died less than forty-eight hours later was that the suite of rooms that was to be her home was an ugly color. I would have to repaint.

This sounds hideous in the telling but this was my mother attitude in most things. She knew I was there. She had been a registered nurse and she was certainly fully aware that whole day of what was going on around her. She did not want to be in that hospital, but she couldn't get herself out. I did. She hated that as much as she needed it. Complaining about the paint was actually her acknowledgement of what I had done. It was no loving hug.

I would like to say that the cases that I have heard through the years are all the loving hug variety, but the plain truth is they are not. The moral of the story here, is that your loved one may not show you the depth of feeling you need as you are facing this change in circumstances, this change that makes you feel as though you have not done enough.

I ask you one question: Would your loved one have been able to live as comfortably as he or she has for the time you have been care for them if you had not been there? If the answer is NO, you have done a great job, mistakes and all. You may not be getting loving hugs but your loved one knows he/she is not alone. You are there.

Do your best to lay your guilt aside as you consider this change in care giving locations. If you must, revisit your feelings later, either alone or with a counselor. For now, clarity of mind and a very realistic view of your care giving situation will make this change process a great deal easier for you and ultimately for the one for whom you are caring. There are steps to be taken here that will help you make an informed choice.

Consult with your loved one's physician. Discuss your issues and concerns fully, especially any physical or behavioral changes. Ask for care suggestions. In my experience, not all doctors feel comfortable offering advice. If you have one of these, don't worry there are other sources.

Take some time to consider what you would like for your loved one. In many ways you know your relative best. Your opinion matters. There are times when an immediate decision must be made. At least give yourself a few hours to think.

A word of caution here: Relatives and friends who often have had little or nothing to do with the care of your loved one may suddenly appear out of the woodwork with all kinds of comments. 'You should have done this. You should have done that. I know just the place. You just want to put them somewhere. That place is too far away for me to visit. It's too expensive.' I have heard all of the above and those are just the nicer comments.

Example: My 92-year-old father-in-law was having mini strokes. My husband, his father and his father's doctor decided among themselves a nursing home was the proper choice. (In those days, assisted living was just getting started and not available everywhere.) My father-in-law had remarried at 85 to a delightful lady who had no problems that we knew of that would require her to follow her husband to the nursing home. Her family had other ideas. I received a nasty phone call, complete with four letter words, from one of her relatives, demanding that we put Papa Clary's wife in the home with him. I refused and tried to explain neither my husband nor had any power to do such a thing. He was not pleased and was very vocal about my refusal. I hung up on him.

What does your loved one want for his or her future? I hope you have already discussed this but if you have not and your relative is mentally aware enough, discuss the situation with them as openly as you can. Be honest. Listen and hear what is being said to you. Remember, no matter how many decisions you have made for them to this point, consider what changing locations really means to them.

Maybe it is moving out of his or her home to yours. Or moving out of yours to assisted living or nursing home. Everything from the walls to how often you see each other is changed. Talk about the choices, what can be and what can't. And why? Just because the body is deteriorating does not mean the mind is.

If at all possible, make the choice together. There are so many reasons for this approach. The most important to me, both as a care giver and one who will one day pass through this stage, the aging person, one who is mentally capable of understanding the situation, has a right to decide the course of his or her life. Aging should not steal your right of choice.

Another reason to share the responsibility is for your sake. You must live with yourself when your loved one is no longer with you. If a decision is made with them, you know you chose what they wanted. You are less likely to spend months maybe even years asking yourself if you chose rightly.

Now that you have made a choice, involve your loved one in the actual decision of which place is best. In the case of a relative who has the mobility and the desire to see the new location, do some preliminary investigation yourself to narrow down a few choices. Then take them to visit each facility. Pay attention to verbal and physical reactions on your relative's side and the care facility. Most likely you will know your own favorite. Example: My father-in-law was well aware that living in his home was no longer possible for him. My husband and I had created a suite for him in the house we lived in at the time. He was very aware that we wanted him to come to us, including his wife who was not my husband's mother. We all got along well but David and I had two very small children with medical issues. Because he was a loving man and a good father who had always taken care of his family, he refused to be a burden, his words never ours.

Because we could not budge him on his choice, I did the research and took him to see the places I thought the best of the group which were close to our home. We chose together.

His wife did not go. Her family came with no warning to us and took her away. If they had not left some luggage behind and had to call us to send it to them, it might have turned into a very bizarre situation. We were her care givers in a sense since she was living in our father-in-law's home. Although she was perfectly capable of taking care of herself, we continued to check on her on a regular basis. If she had gone missing, we certainly would have contacted her relatives but as they were traveling, we would not have gotten anyone. Considering her age, there was a very real possibility we would have called the police. Her four-letter word relative would not have been pleased.

Now, you have placed your relative in the new location. No matter how complete the list was that you used to collect all that he or she would need in the new home, things usually get missed. Also, both you and your loved one will want to see each other, you to be sure your relative is content and he or she to assure himself that you won't just leave him alone day after day and week after week. I didn't try to establish a routine the first few months. In many ways, this transition was harder than the full-time care giving had been. The first days were the most difficult. I was a stay at home working mom. I had left instructions with the care facility to call me if my father-in-law needed anything. (Remember, this was in the days before cell phones). First, it was his favorite windbreaker, then a shirt that had been in the wash and none of us noticed. His favorite after shave was almost gone. The list was varied. For a while I popped in every day for a visit and a list. My husband was working and at school at the time, so his visits weren't as often, mostly just on the weekends.

We were fortunate that I could work from home and take care of the issues. For a working care giver, this transition is many times more difficult. The reassurance visits seem to eat up time and often the care giver is simply worn out with all the demands that have increased to the point the relocation was necessary at all. I wish I could say there is a solution here. There isn't unless you can tap a relative or friend to step in for you while you take a well-earned break. However, since that relative or friend hasn't stepped up to the plate before now, the chances aren't that great. Count on making many trips in the first few weeks. Either you or your partner if you have one, will get a break when things settle down, but relocation is often worse than what you had.

Now, let's talk about the actual living arrangements that your loved one has left behind. If it is a house and it is not rented, you are probably going to be packing up a lifetime of things with an eye to selling the property. If the finances will stand it, I recommend putting furniture, memorabilia etc. in storage until you have had some time to recuperate from the demands that have been made on you and your life. It is too easy here to just pick and choose just to get the job done. Once something special is trashed or sold it is too late to get it back. Worse, if your loved happens to remember and want a special vase, a picture or even a frame, and you have disposed of it, what are either of you going to feel?

Make sure you mark all the boxes. I put a packing sheet in a plastic bag on the side of each box. I don't like unboxing and digging for something I need. And in the case of something small I have a better shot at finding the item in the first box rather the last of fifty.

If the finances won't stand the storage fees or you simply want to get the chore off your list of things to do, packing becomes something you need to do as efficiently as possible. Here are some tips. If you have relatives involved and they are cooperative, rope them in to help. Set up an area for each, including yourself. Work together in the same area. Pick up an item, you don't want it, hold it up and everyone can and choose. This sounds so simple that you are probably shaking your head wondering if I think you are dumb or something. I don't. It just that most people in this situation split up. "I'll take the bedroom; you take the living room. We'll get done faster." No, you won't. You'll spend your time running back and forth with some item in hand to find out if it is wanted. You also won't be using your time very well and a two-day job will turn into three or more. Have a donation pile and a trash bag. If it isn't fit for you to wear or use don't donate. Make a list of what goes in the donation pile. That is tax deductible. In a full house this can be quite a benefit.

Once the house is cleared, it must be cleaned. Clean houses sell better. Depending on finances and time, a cleaning service is a choice possibility. Also, invest in some pleasant air fresheners. Closed up houses, especially old ones, don't always smell good. Again, you are trying to get top dollar for the property. Every tip helps. If you are using a realtor, ask for advice on staging. In some cases, depending on the condition of the furniture, it may be to your advantage to leave things in the house. It may even be possible to include the items in the sale.

If your relative has been living in a rental, your main concern will be the furniture, assuming home was an unfurnished rental, and personal items. You will need to close out the rental and get any deposits back. Be sure to document the condition of the unit with pictures. This will come in handy if there are deposits for damage involved. Also, most units require cleaning before settling any deposit issues. If the finances can handle it, a cleaning service takes the chore off your lists. If not, cleaning supplies and cleaning just became a fact of your life.

If your loved one has been living with you, you will be looking at the remnants of their life in your home. Everything from 'I don't want to deal with this, I don't have the time to deal with this or I don't need to deal with this is will run through your head'. In many ways this part of all the various living arrangements in which I was a direct care giver or indirect one, seems to be the hardest for me. I have been fortunate in that I didn't need the living space immediately in all cases. I had the luxury of being able to shut the door on the space until I had the time and the heart to dismantle what had been created for my loved one and repurpose the area back into my home. I needed that break from my loved one moving out and clearing out their occupation time with me. I needed it because I tired from the long-term care giving and the relocation. I also needed the break because it was hard to face the fact that my loved one wouldn't be with me much longer. I took the time I needed to adjust.

However, it is possible you have a much more immediate need for your space. If financially possible, I highly recommend getting help. For one thing, you won't be facing the task alone. It may be harder than you think. Relief often figures in this equation. I certainly felt it every time. The first time, I felt guilty for months. How could I be glad my relative was someone else's responsibility? That I could just take a deep breath and stop for a minute? That I could get a decent night of sleep without half listening for a voice calling out for help?

There are more thoughts than these few. Every one of them is very real and very true. Love doesn't make the crisis center you have been living in any less true. So, as you are moving out furniture and clothes and little trinkets, keep in mind your loved one isn't the only one facing a huge change. You are too. And more, you are now going to have to live without them in your life in the not too distant future.

More, as the care giver, you will be walking through the coming months and possibly years, if you are fortunate depending on the circumstances, knowing that you soon you will be handling the final arrangements. You have done all you can firsthand. Now you must share the task with strangers. For many care givers this is harder than mere words can convey. Get help if you need it for this stage. Many care facilities have counselors for you and your loved one. Use them. It is hard to shock a counselor in this situation. Most have heard it all and seen more. Also, the more you understand about yourself and what you are doing with, the better able you will be to be there for your relative.

CHAPTER THIRTEEN

HOSPICE

Hospice. The very word rarely creates a moderate reaction. Usually I hear either fear or heartfelt gratitude. First, let's discuss what Hospice is. It is not government. This a private organization that relies on donations, community support and volunteers for most of its services. Some services are unique to certain areas so not all Hospice are exactly the same. But all Hospice share the same basic services. They are there when death is close, hence the fear so many attributes to it. They are there with physical care giving, in the home, in the hospital if necessary, in their own care facility or even in nursing homes in some areas.

They are there for critical care, a 24-hour commitment to the family and to the loved one when death is eminent. They are there with counselors before during and after your relative has passed. They are there with equipment, medications and personnel to make care giving possible in the home instead of a care facility or hospital.

After much thought, I have chosen to create this chapter using examples of my own care giving interaction with Hospice. It is easy to use words to describe this organization. Anyone with a computer can certainly check it out on the web, but a firsthand, no frills recounting of what it does when needed would count more with me if I was facing the need for Hospice. So, the following are three stories from my perspective as a care giver.

As recounted earlier, my mother was in the hospital. Treatment to return her home was not occurring and the doctor involved was not interacting with my family as we needed. After talking with the nurses and one of specialists on the case, I decided to call in Hospice. Within fifteen minutes of making the request of the case manager, the Hospice case worker arrived. She went over my options. I explained I had a very real feeling that if my mother wasn't moved out the hospital that day, she very well might die in the one place she did not want to be. Many people might have brushed my worry off. I wasn't referring to her care in the hospital l. I was referring to a deep feeling she was very close to death. I have to add here, that I have been closely involved with a number of family members at this time of life. I had discovered I could often tell when the time was approaching. I am not sure why she appeared to believe me, especially since my mother was in rare form, driving everyone nuts trying to keep her happy.

She simply nodded and turned to the hospital administrator's assistant and outlined what she would need. The hospital administrator was working on getting my mother discharged by a doctor who was managing to hide from all of us. She turned to me and explained my mother would need certain equipment her Hospice area couldn't provide simply because all of theirs was in use. She would pull in the needed items from surrounding Hospice areas. It took just about twelve hours to bring in a hospital bed, respiratory equipment and a person to instruct me in use, special foods (these I got with a list from the nurse), bedside commode, tray table, a nurse with a medication box for my refrigerator and medical transport to bring my mother home at approximately 10:30 pm that same night. We had everything we needed to duplicate the care she had been receiving in the hospital. She knew she was home.

By the next day, about midday she did not. She died the following morning at about 8:30 am. I only had to make one phone call to Hospice. They had a nurse in the way in minutes. She handled everything, calling the funeral home and readying my mother for transport. She was there to talk if we needed it while we waited. To arrange for pick-up of all the equipment that had just been brought in so that my father would not have to stay in the room looking at the equipment at such a time. She even helped us remove most of it to the garage so that only the bed remained until the truck could get there.

The following day, Hospice followed up with a call to see if we needed a grief counselor either for my family, the care givers, or my brother family which included children. For the first year we received constant monthly contacts offering support. That could have been declined at will. I did not simply because there were so many of us to consider and someone might need more help than I or anyone could give. It was helpful to just know that help was there.

My best friend of thirty plus years was in ICU and her family was with her. I didn't live in the area and I had called to find out how she was. After being assured that she was well but was remaining in ICU, I hung up the phone. Again, I was feeling as though 'fine' was not an accurate description. I talked it over with my husband and we decided I would go to visit her. The trip was a five-hour drive. When I arrived, her family was kind enough to get special permission for me to see my friend. The breathing tube she had been on had just been taken out. She could barely mouth the words but somehow, she had the strength to push out 'I want to go home'. The nurse had come in with me and heard her. After promising I would do my best to get her what she wanted, the two of us walked out together. The family was in the waiting area, taking a much need break. The nurse indicated the family was aware that my friend was not going to get better. She seemed to think that they were aware of how close the time was. I knew how loved my friend was and I knew from personal experience how hard what they were facing was.

I went to find her son and told him what his mother wanted. He confirmed the information with his mother. She was certainly lucid enough to make her own decisions. Hospice was called in to arrange for the relocation. Unfortunately, my friend went into a coma and relocating wasn't possible. Instead, Hospice brought her home to my friend. The ICU room had a small cart with coffee brewing, snacks and drinks on ice. A small boom box with a selection of tapes if we wanted music for ourselves or my friend, a Bible, an offer of a minister to sit with us, The drapes were drawn and the door closed and draped and the nurses, slowly and quietly at intervals, disconnected the machines that were keeping my friend with us. We were there for five hours. We spent the time telling each of special moments with Edith. Her son had great stories. Her oldest friend even stopped by as if for a chat. It wasn't home but it wasn't the sterile, regimented environment of a hospital either. When the moment arrived, we were all with her. She was not alone with strangers. Hospice made that possible.

The last story concerns my husband. He had stage four lung cancer. Although he fought for a year, despite his strength and the best efforts of his doctors he was losing the battle. He was in a care facility after surgery on his hip for a cancerous tumor. I could see that we didn't have much longer and asked for Hospice. Normally, the doctor should be the one to make the request. But as you can see from the examples above that is not always the case. I explained my concerns to his nurse, and she arranged for the case worker to come in about 10 am. By three that afternoon, the equipment needed to support my husband in a home setting arrived and shortly after that so did my husband. He was so weak, but he had the strength to lift his head and look around. Talking was almost impossible for him by then but he said, "I'm home."

A nurse arrived to assess everything to make sure we had all we needed. In the process of the assessment, I discovered another wonderful thing about Hospice. It had a program called critical care. The nurse explained the service was only for one 24-hour period. As the sole caregiver I was worn out. I doubted my ability to be as careful with the pain medications as I usually was, and I had no experience with liquid morphine. My husband wanted to be home and I wanted that for him whatever the cost to me or our finances. The 24-hour period would give me the time to decide how to handle the hours or days beyond that. I accepted Hospice's help. What I didn't know at the time, was no one expected my husband to last that day. He was with me for four more days. I had a nurse the whole time. Every day, an assessment was made, and the care was extended one more day.

David had the medical care he needed to make his last days as comfortable as possible and I had the support I needed, as I never had before. There was nurse right with us to make sure that as David's pain escalated, the medication was increased. His comfort was paramount. Hospice gave us that security, that compassion, that skilled caring in our own home.

This is what Hospice can and does do every day. The medical professional is focused on preserving life at all costs. Machines, medications, procedures, and surgeries all play a valuable part in the aging process. Hospice focuses on the patient first, last and always in my opinion. The patient's comfort, needs and wishes are the starting and ending points. When Hospice entered any situation that involved my loved ones or any one of my extended family of friends' loved ones, the doctors and hospitals stepped back. The focus changed from fighting a losing battle for life and engaging in a winning battle for grace in leaving life. I have never regretted calling in Hospice. There have been tiny errors here and there. No group of people no matter how wonderful and dedicated can do something so important without a bobble or two but where my loved ones were concerned, those mistakes didn't matter at all. Everyone in my family and in the families of friends was where he or she wanted to be, in the way he or she wanted to be and with those who mattered the most to him or her.

CHAPTER FOURTEEN

WHEN YOUR CHILD COMES HOME TO LIVE

Not all care giving situations fall into the care of an aging loved one. Many of the issues already discussed will apply in the situations we will be discussing. However, many care giving arrangements have special needs and problems. I will attempt to address some of these here. Again, this book is not about having all the answers. It is about spawning ideas and possible solutions to some of the issues you may be encountering.

CHILDREN Unfortunately, it is a growing trend in this country for grandparents, aunts, uncles or siblings to be taking care of children that are not their own. With fractured families, deaths and economic pressures, a parent, working or retired, may suddenly find him/herself with a child and their children at the door needing a home. Or a daughter marries and brings hubby home to live at your house while they save for their own. Or a child dies and grandmother and grandfather take in one or more children because the father isn't available or able to be the parent.

Yanking the covers over your head and praying that what you are looking at is only a nightmare and you will wake up and everything will be just as it was won't work. It isn't a nightmare. It's reality in the twenty-first century.

If the situation is an adult child, with or without a spouse or partner, needing a home, you have the ability to sit down with the individual and discuss what you want, need and expect. So many people with whom I have come in contact with this problem don't discuss but react. The adult child pops into the allotted room and mom becomes mom again and dad becomes dad. However, the adult child does not become the child again. This is where the problems begin, in my opinion. Suddenly, Mom has double or triple the laundry and cleaning. Meals are bigger and messier. The electric bill increases the hot water decreases. Dad needs help and the kid isn't ever around. He isn't saving money if he is out all night. She isn't saving money if she is always at the mall or with the girls after work at the local hang out. Add a spouse or partner neither of you know or even one you think you do know, and the problems escalate. When I was faced with this situation, when my daughter married and brought her husband home to our house, I tried the sit down and discuss method. I had already learned my lesson about guessing and reacting when caring for my husband's family, so don't give me credit for being smart here. I just try to learn from my mistakes. Respect is the key here. Respect for your needs and theirs will make living together smoother and more rewarding.

Here are the points we addressed. We'll start with adult children, with a spouse or partner.

Establish the relationship Sharing space sounds simple but it isn't even under the best of conditions. When stranger is added, such as a spouse or partner, the problems can escalate without you even realizing it. Add to that equation, one member of the pair is your child who is now an adult and it is easy to see problems can occur.

Establishing a rapport from the start will ease the way for any problem. Talking to your child may be your go to but think of the spouse or partner too. Leaving him or her out is not going to feel good from the new addition's point of view. Try talking together in a relaxed atmosphere, over dinner or lunch maybe. Outline your thoughts on the new living arrangements, the crosses in schedules or needs, the compromises you are willing to make to ease the way.

I lead with what I am willing to do first rather than demand someone else do something first. Again, I started working with others in my home or theirs at a very early age. Offering what I could do was the go-to for me. I discovered through the years this approach made an easier opening, a less confrontational beginning to any discussion where compromises were needed.

Example: My daughter lived at home in a mother-in-law suite. She met and married a delightful man in less than seven weeks. She asked us if she could continue to live at home until they could save some money for a place of their own. We agreed. Although we liked her new husband very much, we didn't know him at all well. Both worked. Both had cars as did we. No one had the same work schedule. Needless to say, our drive was a minefield for all of us when anyone needed to get his or her out. We all gathered on the porch one evening after a morning of who moves what so who can get to work. Everyone had a soda or tea and all of us were looking at the cars and trucks filling the drive. Everyone had an idea, and everyone was ready to ditch the current arrangement. It didn't take long for all of us to agree on a spot for each vehicle. This area of the yard was big enough if I didn't mind losing a little grass. The guys went out to move the vehicles and my daughter and I decided spaghetti would make a great dinner.

Whatever space you allot to your son/daughter, treat it with respect. In other words, if you have given him or her a bedroom and a bath, don't enter the area especially if the door is closed without knocking and waiting for permission to enter. Yes, I know it is your house, but for the time being, you have given them a portion to call home. How would you feel if someone barged in without asking?

Arrange common appliance usage schedules. Share a washer and/or dryer with another couple without a schedule and see how well that works for you. It is almost a guarantee of a fight among dirty clothes. Don't forget to consider the hot water supply in this discussion. If everyone in the household works, try to arrange showers so no one is yelling "What happened to the hot water?" In our house, it was my husband who boomed that out at 6 am if I happened to forget.

Sharing a kitchen can be another trouble spot. Again, talk and listen. Shared meals are not always the best answer. If you are a person who hates dishes on the counter or in the sink, make that clear in a nice but firm way. Don't wait until you are looking at a mess when you haven't even had your coffee yet in the morning. The chances of you being nice then are not great. Talk about food purchases if you are sharing a refrigerator or pantry. Don't poach without asking and discuss that as well.

Sharing entertainment space Indoor and outdoor space falls in this category. Just because you have others living with you does not mean you want to give up a social life. Discuss your needs in this area, a social or committee meeting once a week in your home, the Super Bowl party you planned before you increased your household. Your friends aren't necessarily theirs nor theirs yours. Are you going to allow them to entertain in your home and if so how? Address their needs and yours as fairly as you can.

Depending on your situation, you can have more points than these. Make a list. Talk to your spouse if you have one and get his/her opinion before you begin any discussion. And, if problems arise, discuss with your spouse first before approaching the other couple. A united front in these situations takes one more possible problem off the table. Families are a delight for many and a bane of existence for the rest. Try to remember, even in the best of family's issues do arise. You want to end this shared living arrangement still enjoying the same relationship with your son or daughter. Who knows? It may even be better.

Next, let's look at a son or daughter returning home with a child or children. If the spouse is with your offspring, the information above still applies. However, children had a new dimension.

Children are noisy. The best-behaved child in the universe is, generally, not quiet. Depending on the lifestyle of your household, this could be a major issue from hour one. If you work from home, it is not just an issue it is an ISSUE. Lay the ground rules out clearly and the reasons for them. Your offspring may know them but not the spouse. If the children are old enough include them in the conversation.

Create an area where the children may be noisy and messy without involving the whole household. When space is limited as it probably will be with the influx of people this is going to need some creative thinking. But children need room, a place to play, to bounce around and just be kids. All of you are having to make compromises to make this shared arrangement work. Children don't necessarily understand that or even remember it.

If you have a garage, maybe the car can live outside for the duration and you can make a play area inside for the kids. Heating/cooling may be an issue and, of course, making sure the area is safe and secure is a must. However, a little creative thinking makes for better relations among you all.

Sleeping space Living space is at a premium in most situations like this. Having children bunk on the floor in the family room for a sleepover is one thing. Having that for an indeterminate length of time is another. It won't work for you or them. More, the children will feel less because, even a little guy can figure out everyone has a real bed but him. Again, being creative is going to be helpful. Twin beds, pull-out beds, and couches that turn into beds are all options. Whatever you do, try to emphasize the positive for the child. Example: "Look, your bed is special. You don't have to make it like I do. You can just push it under the big bed, and no one will see it. It's your secret. And best of all you don't have that chore on your list. I wish I could do that with mine."

Shared living arrangements make imposing easier If you are the type who doesn't like babysitting children, make your feelings clear from the beginning. Maybe you don't mind helping out with this chore if someone has to work overtime or attend a special meeting. But just because you are home and your son/daughter wants to go out and has no idea when he/she will return, may not be at all to you taste. Make that clear before the situation arises. The grandparent manual does not have a rule that says every grandparent just loves being an unpaid babysitter who has no idea when the parents will return.

Children are a joy for most parents and grandparents but often, especially in times of crisis, we can forget the impact of that crisis on the young. The chances are you won't get ahead of every difficulty, but you will get many. Because you take the time to try, the children aren't just tag-alongs in the crisis. They are important and loved to the best of your ability. They may not understand it now, but they will when they are older. And maybe the hard choices you make will be passed on to a generation you may not get to meet.

Pets Pets are often family members who cannot be left behind just because there is a crisis. If your family member is bringing a pet into your house, especially if you have pets of your own, sit down and discuss how you are going to handle the new arrival. If the pet is house trained and you don't mind it running loose in the home, there isn't much to change as long as your own pets have no problem with the newcomer.

However, if your pets do have a problem so do you and your family member. Don't automatically assume all is well, especially if you are leaving the animals at home alone while everyone works. Take a little time to acclimate the animals to each other. A traveling cage is a good way for the newcomer to get acquainted until you see how the animal family relates. A baby gate across a doorway works well in containing the newcomer and still allows the residents to stop by to visit.

Consider the feeding station if it is an indoor pet. Many animals have difficulty eating together. Staggering the feeding times and separating your pets from theirs may solve the issue.

CHAPTER FIFTEEN

GRANDPARENTS RAISING GRANDCHILDREN

This next section is addressing a tragedy, a parent losing a child with children in death. I cannot think of a worse situation for a parent to face. The grief is so huge and so consuming that life after is a distant if even thinkable possibility. When this tragedy is accompanied by children who have lost a mother or father and now are going to be living with you, grief is buried under the burden of just coping with each step in the processes of burial, clearing the child's home and taking belongings to storage or your own home and, most demanding of all, caring for the grieving grandchildren.

Because I wanted this book to be about real situations and solutions, I chose to ask a friend of mine (forty-three years of sharing life's problems) to give me her input on this aspect of care giving. She is living this life with all of its complications, fears, doubts, angers, laughter, tears and frustrations. In order to fully understand and show the heavy demands in this situation, I asked my friend, Cindy, for her permission to give some details of this life changing tragedy.

Every story will be different, more terrible, more complicated by finances, lack of family to support, shorter or longer depending on circumstances. This is just one story that changed the future of a comfortable retirement into instant parenthood.

On February 13, 2011, my friend and her husband, lost their daughter. Her death came out of a simple household accident that could have happened to anyone. The daughter thought the accident minor and went to a friend's house for a party. She was early and feeling a little sore from the fall she had taken, she laid down for a bit until time for the party. When she didn't appear, someone checked on her and found her unresponsive. The police were called. My friend and her husband were notified, and the nightmare began. Christy had two sons, eight and fifteen. My friend's second thought was for them. They went straight to Christy's house to pick up the children.

In less than two hours, Cindy and her husband, sixty-three and sixty-seven respectively, turned from grandparents to parents. There was no preparation for the children or the grandparents. There was no manual for the legal issues that popped up like popcorn. There was no pamphlet on being questioned by the police and living through their daughter's life being scrutinized. No one explained what to do with an eight-year-old who needed constant reassurance and clung to Cindy's side through those first days while his grandparents dealt with the myriad of details of their daughter's death, investigation, autopsy and funeral. A mother and father's grief was buried under the life thrust upon them. They coped. What choice was there? The remaining family gathered around them. Christy was a twin, so her sister's grief was complicated by that, from birth, intimate sibling connection. Their grown son made arrangements to relocate his job to be available to help.

Every situation is different, and every state has its own laws that may come into play with the change in your life. For the ease of reading and finding what may be important issues for you I have created a simply worded list. Nothing can blunt the edges and tears in the heart of grief. Nothing can help those moments when you want to lay your head down and just cry but can't because a grieving child needs you. Counseling, family and friends may be there, but you are the one who feels the loss to the depths of your being. There is no time limit. Nor is there any perfect way to grieve. Screaming might help but the grief is still there when you are done. So, I hope, as you cope with this new lifestyle you neither sought nor wanted, that someone, somewhere tells you, and often, just how wonderful you are for shredding your life and rebuilding it for the sake of these children you love.

As much as possible, according to age and situation, be honest and forthcoming with the child. Remember, as much as your situation has changed, his or hers has too. Both of you are grieving. Make the conversations as comfortable as possible. Handing out orders is hard in any circumstance. Try softer approaches if possible, a meal, an outing. Set down the basics of the moment. Details can wait if possible until either the situations appear, or two sides have had some time to settle into the new life a little.

Be prepared for fears in the child, both already established and new ones. Their world and everything they knew is now gone and their new world is being established. They wonder if they will picked-up on time and no longer want to stay home alone. Any fear which may appear irrational is mostly normal and eases with time. Pets bring a great deal of comfort if possible. There is also counseling available through a referral from a physician to a professional. Schools, churches and Hospice are other sources for counseling. There is help. Pride need not be an issue here. Most of us are not equipped to handle this kind of complex situation. Counselors can offer support to you and your child.

Try to establish the new family unit as quickly as possible. One simple way is having dinner together each evening so that there is time to talk and relate to each other in this new way.

The new family needs to be as cohesive as possible ASAP so that there is a naturalness about the relationship. The grandparent is often accustomed to having the child in the home, spoiling them rotten, sugaring them up and returning them to the parent with a satisfied smirk. No longer! Now, you are the parent, and they are home. The last thing you need is a sugared up, hyperactive or whiney child to manage.

Any remaining family may wish to be involved with the child. If there is another set of grandparents, some disagreements can arise. Family situations are minefields in the best of times. If at all possible, try to work with the other family members to come agreement on visiting and outing for the child. Adults are grieving but the children are not and should not be methods or objects for dealing with that grief. Grief is difficult from an adult perspective but from a child's it can be even more difficult. The child is looking to his or her family for support, comfort and security. Familial arguments will not help the child feel secure or comfortable.

Grandparents raising grandchildren is so common that most cities have groups with that name. This group is an amazing source of information and comfort. Many grandparents have already been doing this job for quite a while and have tremendous helpful experience to share. If a lawyer is needed and unaffordable, these groups often have lawyers who are dedicated to help for a nominal fee, if a fee at all. There are monthly meetings and social events that include the child. Usually there is no problem that arises that someone is this group has not solved.

Custody of the child is critical and immediate. The child cannot receive medical treatment or be enrolled in school without it. If possible, a family lawyer is the best advocate. It's not cheap by any means but, depending on the circumstances, that lawyer will go to the wall to complete the custody paperwork. Even then, the papers will say "Temporary". Unless there is a renegade relative seeking custody, the temporary custody agreement takes care of everything.

Make several copies of all legal papers and keep a permanent file. The page with the seal is not necessary for most entities so many expensive copies need not be purchased.

Make copies of everything! The parent's death certificate, occasionally the parent's birth certificate is also required so copy it as well, the child's birth certificate, the child's Social Security card, the insurance card. If possible, create a file on the computer and keep everything in it so a new copy can be created at a moment's notice. This may sound like overkill, but it eventually is a great source of comfort and convenience to know all the information is safe and accessible.

Once the custody is established, then and only then, can the grandparent be appointed the representative or agent to receive the child's Social Security. The money received will be retroactive to the date of the parent's death. Coming as a complete surprise was the letter received a year later from the Social Security demanding to know how the money was spent! If the grandparent is absconding with the money, this is understandable but, at the time, when one feels the land under his feet is finally becoming established, the letter feels like an insult. Also, if money has been placed in a savings or college fund, the letter the following year has added the previously saved money to the new yearly total and more explanations are necessary.

Keep good records. A separate bank account should be set up for the child and the grandparent. All monthly statements must be kept and, if banking online, print out that statement and make a note of the reason for all expenditures. It is handy to bank online so that necessary funds can be transferred to the grandparent's account for monthly expenses.

DO NOT FEEL GUILTY about spending the money for clothing, school expenses, special food treats or entertainment. That is what the money is meant to do. The grandparent does not need to have her monthly finances stretched beyond comfort if at all possible.

Also, if the finances will stretch to it, set up a 529 college account. If only a small portion is deposited every month, it grows quickly, especially if the child is young and the money can be placed in a higher risk investment category. For the older child, it is smarter to place most of the funds in a money market type category 529 so that what is invested will not be lost through the fluctuation of the market. As the investing grandparent, the decision of which category to place the funds in is entirely up to you.

As high school graduation approaches, there are many scholarships and grants offered for a child who has lost a parent. Research will be needed here to find the appropriate ones for your child. School advisors can be a great source of information as well as the internet.

Generally, grandparents do not have a health insurance plan which will cover a newly inherited child. Obamacare may change this but for now, the state's offer a plan at a reasonable cost. It is basically a "KIDCARE" plan and depending on the amount of the Social Security the child receives; it may fall into the "KIDCARE Medicaid" category. Almost all pediatricians accept these plans. These plans have to be renewed annually so be prepared and apply early to avoid extra stress.

The cost of the plan is based ONLY on the child's Social Security amount. The state has no right to the amount of the grandparent's Social Security, retirement pensions, savings, or property ownership.

Remember you have temporary custody not adoption status. If you are considering permanent custody or adoption, other factors and requirements will apply. Legal advice is a must here, for your sake and the child's. There are groups who address these situations and many offer legal contacts who work for reduced rates or no cost depending on circumstances. Adoption, for instances, removes a number of benefits which would otherwise be available for the child.

Phone calls will often have to be made to the state insurance agency. Keep all numbers in a file for quick reference. Each child has a number and there is a family account number. Also be prepared to be 'on hold' for a very long time and often, the person answering is difficult to understand.

In our situation, we pay $15 a month for the insurance which is not Medicaid. This can be paid online with a credit card. Primary Care Pediatrician's fee is $0. Referrals to specialists are required and their fee is $5. Also, covered prescriptions are $5. It is comforting to know that medical care is affordable and available.

Finally, time passes and actually much faster than expected. The wounds of grief, though still and always present, are not as raw. On a particularly retrospective day, the grandparent can sit back, witness the progress and accomplishments of the child and realize that though they wish everything was different, they are doing a good job. There is a lot to be said for age and experience. A grandparent knows how quickly a child grows to adulthood and how truly unimportant in the grand scheme of life that bad grade is, or the cluttered bedroom or the dirty face and clothing. They realize the child appreciates the bold truth when asking a question and though the truth doesn't always set us free, it eases the pressure of the shackles. The phrase 'this too shall pass' not only becomes clearer, it becomes a mantra. The phrase 'this is not my first rodeo' becomes almost comical and whoever said 'laughter is the best medicine' was probably raising grandchildren. Despite the tears, the fears, the angst, the anger and even, finally, the resumption of happiness and normalcy—-LIFE DOES GO ON.

Of course, not all grandparents have the raising of their grandchildren due to death of the parent. In today's world of fractured families, the grandparent may have to step in because of legal issues such as imprisonment or child neglect or the parent may simply give up the child. Each of these issues come with a whole basket of problems for the grandparent. It is important that the grandparent understand his or her rights and obligations in caring for the child. Financial assistance Social Security may be possible. Insurance help. Legal protection for you or the child or both may be necessary. Legal help and advice here is critical for all your sakes. There are resources for legal help. If you are dealing with the law enforcement community seek information from them on sources. Schools are also possible sources of information. The internet if you have access to it is another. Churches are another.

CHAPTER SIXTEEN

CARE GIVING LIST

At first glance, this chapter may seem like a repeat of information already scattered in different sections of this book. It is. However, because I wanted to create an easy to read and use manual of sorts, I thought a list of basic points in one place would make a difficult task just a little simpler. Whether you are caring for your loved one in your home or theirs, there are certain things that it pays to monitor. Below, is a list and the reasons for the attention. This is by no means a list that you, depending on circumstances, won't have items of your own to add but it is a list that hits some spots very easily missed in day to day living.

Hygiene Don't assume your relative takes care of all hygiene issues on a daily basis. Memory or simple discomfort may make your loved one choose to skip labor intensive things, from their point of view, such as a shower or tooth brushing. No, you don't have to ask them directly like a warden. Simply ease into the bath and check the bath towel and the toothbrush. If neither is wet, it is a good bet, neither was used. Missing a day once in a while is generally not going to be an issue, but a regular lack of care is these areas will create skin and dental problems which can, in extreme cases, require a doctor's attention and possibly even hospitalization.

Skin Care Be aware of changes in skin health especially if your loved one has diabetes or any disease which causes major changes in the skin. Rashes left untreated can become infected. Blotches that change color or texture can be cancerous at worst or need a simple treatment at best. Unclean skin area, especially those that are subject to chafing or rubbing can create sores. Staph doesn't just exist in hospitals and it is difficult to heal and treat even in a young person.

Toenails and Foot Care This is especially important if your loved one has diabetes. Check with your relative's doctor and his insurance to find out the qualifications for a podiatrist. Most insurances, in the case of diabetics, allows for regular visit to this specialist. But even with regular visit it won't be daily attention. As one ages, bending over to the feet or getting the feet in a position for trimming nails is harder if not impossible. Nails become over long and can scratch or cut limbs, catching on sheets, rugs as trip hazards or just be rip from the toe entirely to bleed everywhere. Equally the places between toes are nice breeding grounds for sores and infections. If your loved one is a woman, a pedicure is an easy solution, either the home variety or in a salon. With a male relative the solution might be a little trickier. Be creative if necessary but don't neglect this area. The solutions for problems here can be expensive and time consuming.

Groceries and Foods Even though your relative may be doing his or her own shopping, keep an eye on the pantry supplies and the cleanliness of the refrigerator. Expiration dates on products, leftovers in the frig for more than a few days are all sources of risk. Again, being a warden is not the answer. Checking can be done subtly as you get a glass of water or a snack. Or simply offer to clean the frig for Mom or Dad to save them the trouble. Since I have always had dogs, I talked my relatives into allowing me to check out the frig for scraps for the guys. It was a good reason for having my nose in the food supplies and my dogs loved me bunches.

Dehydration It is amazing how easy it is for anyone to become dehydrated. Since I have spent most of my adult life in hot South Florida, I was very aware of dehydration as a health risk. In the aging population it is critically important both because of existing health issues and medications but just in general. Check with your loved one's doctor for the fluid intake that should be maintained for health. Then discuss the importance of drinking fluids with your loved one. Make sure there are enough choices to cater to need.

Since I am in the aging sector now, I keep bottled water on hand from the first thing in the morning until I get ready for bed. It not only reminds me to drink, something I have always forgotten even as a kid, but it makes it easy for me to see how many bottles have consumed that day in addition to the fluids with meals.

I also make sure that my relative has water with a flexible straw beside the bed at night. Medications can cause drying of the mouth as can open mouth sleeping. Having water close at hand means better fluid intake as well as lessening the fumbling around in the dark to get to the kitchen.

Bed Care Making a bed is labor intensive for many of the aging population. Because activity is reduced many consider changing linen on a regular unnecessary. Not true. As long as no wound or sore issues are involved, linen should be changed at least once a week, more often if the relative is bed ridden. If you have a question due to your circumstances, check with a nurse either at the doctor's office or the on-call nurse that most insurances provide at no cost.

Check the mattress pad as well. Speaking of the mattress pad, budget allowing, invest in a waterproof one. Accidents do happen. Something as simple as spilling a glass of water on the bed will mean you need a hair dryer to dry the spot or risk your loved one sleeping on damp sheets and mattress. Again, time consuming and annoying. You have enough to do without adding things to the list.

Overall cleaning In your home or theirs, cleaning the living area itself, including windows, floors and furniture is important. In my care giving, I found in my younger years, a good shake down twice a year did the trick without making my wish to scream. However, once I hit 55, I decided I would rather pay someone to come in twice a year and do the big stuff like windows and carpets and turn out kitchen cabinets. Yes, it cost a bit but when I looked at the hours and wear & tear on my body, I felt it was worth it. Not all budgets will stand this cost so talking to some of your family members about helping, either financially in hiring someone or sweat equity in helping you, might take some of the burden off you.

Doctor and Dentist Appointments As much as possible, attend appointments with your relative. Keep a list of any concerns you may have and any questions. Get answers you understand and write them down. Any changes in behavior, depression is not uncommon in the aging process, or physical condition should be discussed.

Shopping with your relative Shopping can be fun or a misery. Just popping into a car and zipping to the mall is probably not going to be that easy anymore, especially if your relative has mobility issues. Just loading him or her and the equipment needed for the outing will be time consuming and a challenge.

Depending on the mobility aid involved, a handicap tag may be a real work saver as well as a convenience. Your relative's doctor will be needed to fill out the paperwork for the tag to be issued. These are free but do have to be renewed.

While we are here, let's talk about mobility aids. What they do? What they don't? The equipment aids your loved one but nothing, so far, reproduces the original ease of movement. Try using a cane for two hours and you learn firsthand the answer to both questions. Try using a walker for two hours. Or a wheelchair. Just to get up out of the car and balanced in a parking lot is a challenge. Going through doors is another obstacle. Moving fast is another. I tried all of my relatives' equipment to determine the issues so that I could help if necessary and keep my hands and thoughts to myself if it wasn't. Your loved one is frustrated enough with his or her aging process. A little understanding here makes for a better relationship between you.

Entry into a store is no longer just a simple issue. Inclement weather further complicates the problem. Depending on your loved one and the aid involved, here is a simple example of how to make entry a little easier.

Find a parking place. If you already have a handicap tag, you have a space close to the entrance. If your relative has a wheelchair, you can unload the chair and your loved one is set to go shopping.

If your loved one has a cane or walker, I recommend using one of the motorized carts that most big stores and malls have. In the case of a mall, call ahead to check availability, if you don't already know. You leave the car and go into the store and get one of the motorized carts. Return to the car and your relative takes the cart. No matter how much fun shopping is, it is tiring too, even for the twenty somethings. Also, the cane and walker can be left in the car and out of the way for the expedition.

HINT: Walk with your relative as though he or she was still walking. DO NOT LEAD OR SHOP AND RETURN MULTIPLE TIMES. It's rude and it gives the impression that your loved one is slowing you down or wasting time. Your relative then feels a burden. This is not a good feeling for anyone, no matter the age.

Bathrooms in stores

Traveling-Traveling can be a challenge in spite of the various handicap accessible laws. If you use a travel agent for your travel plans, the agent can check hotels and tour companies for accommodations. If you are booking online, I suggest contacting hotel/motels directly to make sure of room placement, elevator location, loading and unloading areas etc. Here are a few things that make traveling easier.

Where is the entrance? Is it covered? Is it handicap accessible? Older hotels/motels may have separate entrances for handicap. I don't like these and generally steer clear of them. It is a personal preference on my part based on the feelings it evokes in me. I don't like my relatives or friends to feel diminished by the aging they cannot control. A separate handicap entrance tends to do just that. If he/she can't go in the front entrance, I can't either. I find another hotel.

Where are the elevators? Most hotels have them situated close to the desk and the entrance doors.

What kind of flooring? A glossy marble floor in a posh hotel looks fantastic but for someone with a cane and sometimes even with a walker it is a minefield especially in wet weather.

Where is the handicap accessible room? At the end of the hall? Near the elevators?

If your relative has medications that need refrigeration, be sure to check that the room has that feature.

If you are using a tour bus or trolley for sightseeing, does it have handicap accessibility? So far, I haven't encountered one that does not, but it pays to check.

If you are taking your relative to one of the theme parks, motorized carts are available at the entrance but after you have journeyed a good distance in a huge parking lot and possibly even a long walk to the turnstiles to pay your way in. These carts cannot be reserved. It is first come first serve so went there early.

In large cities, it is possible to rent a scooter chair or cart for the duration of your stay. The cart is delivered to your hotel and is returned the same way. The only catch here is that you will need to be staying in a theme park hotel. It is not a requirement of the cart company as much as it is a transport necessity. Having the rental cart is only convenient if you have a ramp in the vehicle you are using for transport. If you are already on the grounds of the theme park, their transport vehicles are handicap accessible and the problem is solved.

Plane travel is relatively easy. Letting the sky cap know you need assistance when you pull at the terminal will ensure a wheelchair will arrive to convey your relative through the inspections and to the departure area. You may have to wait if the terminal is a very busy one.

Train travel. Handicap assistance is also available here as well. Again, check with the station you will be using to confirm.

Ship travel. Confirm handicap arrangements when you make your reservations. Cabins are not always as large as you may need. If in doubt, because you are going to be there for a number of days with no way off, I like measuring out the area in my own house, including furniture. If you can't move around there you won't be able to move around on the boat. Also, if your relative has medications that need refrigeration, check to see how that will be handled.

Documentation Be sure when you travel that you carry documentation with you and keep it in a safe place, on your person is best or a safe. You will need medical insurance cards and numbers, a list of medications and numbers for refills. Medical history, your relative's doctor is a good source for this. Passport, copy of birth certificate and DNR, your loved one's will, health surrogate and power of attorney in case of accident or hospitalization. You cannot speak for your relative if you do not have the legal right to do so. Carry the paperwork.

If you have not already attended to the items above, now would be the time. I highly recommend legal advice. Yes, I know you can do most of this on the internet but what if you don't get it right? When you need it most will probably be the time you find out you should have contacted a lawyer and paid the fee for the documentation to be done by a professional.

Final arrangements. I know you don't want to do this one. Who does? But you will need to discuss with your loved one what he/she wants when their time is complete. If arrangements have not already been made, work with them to make them. It is a difficult task for both of you, but this must be done. You will not want to guess at what your relative might have wanted.

Finally, as always throughout the book, these are suggestions. Your situation may be different. The point of this list is to eliminate trouble and problems for both you and your loved one. Aging takes a toll on all of us, the aging and the care giver. A little thought makes life a lot smoother. I wanted to enjoy, as much as possible, the remaining time I had with my family members. The planning and the forethought gave me that luxury. No, I did not get everything right. But the big stuff, the important stuff for me and mine was there. I wish I had had longer. I didn't.

Life has its own timetable. But I did have fun. My family members died exactly where they wanted to be, in my home or theirs. Only one had to go to a care facility and he chose that route because of the medical care issues. We chose his new home together. Although he lasted only six months, he liked his place, the wide screened porch that opened onto a nature preserve where is could watch the birds and the rabbits play.

Because of them, Grandmother Cook, Grandpop Cook, Uncle Bill, Mama Clary, Papa Clary, Mother, Pop, Edith, and my husband David, this book exists. Because of friends and their needs at this time of life, because of friends of friends and their families, I was able to draw even more experiences in the creating of this manual. Because of all of these lives, I have been able to create a home specifically designed for aging. I live in a place where I can grow old in peace and the knowledge that leaving won't be an issue that my children will have to face.

In an age of space stations and satellites, we have yet to create homes that last a lifetime of changing. We have granite counter tops and stainless-steel appliances in our dream homes, but we don't commonly build our houses in a way to keep those things when we have a walker or a wheelchair as we age. Nor do we build homes that accommodate multi generations with any ease. In my area, the building codes are even stacked against this arrangement in most counties. What is that saying about building a better mousetrap? I would settle just for an improved one. I spent my earning years creating a lifestyle and the minute I retire I am supposed to downsize. Why? Is this the best we can do as we age? I hope not.

ABOUT THE AUTHOR

Why would a traditionally published author, published internationally with over thirty books in more than twenty languages and two lifetime achievement awards just to name few accolades, choose to self-publish?

If your first answer is that she has lost her mind, my answer is NO!

You'll notice the capital letters. Film stars regularly finance and produce their movies and movies of other stars. Why can't authors choose to produce their books, leaving behind the traditional format for the freedom of writing what the author wants and when the author wants to write?

I haven't lost my mind. I've gained by creative freedom. Writing is more than a career for me. It always has been, from the moment I ran out of books and decided, for my sanity's sake, to write a story while I waited for more books to arrive. A fluke involving another writer who had just started a writing club was my first brush with the machinery that is traditional publishing.

It was supposed to be hard to get an agent. That writer thought I had talent, although she didn't tell me that at the time, and she sent my story to her agent. I sold four books that year.

I discovered that interesting word genre. Darn it. I had to write a certain way. Because I had a 'male' name and only women wrote romances at that time, I had to have a pen name. Because I wrote faster than my home house would publish a single writer, my agent sent my extra stories to other houses. Each wanted a different pen name. Hence, I have multiple pen names.

Lacey Dancer was and is my favorite. It represents a moment in my life when I called a halt to the process of traditional publishing. I was worn out by the rules and requirements. I understood their business model and it does work for publishing in general. It didn't work for me the writer. I wanted to create real people characters, dealing with real problems. Life is too interesting to be reduced to a fairy tale.

After a discussion with my agent, I decided to quit. It wasn't the first time I'd made that decision. She had four of my books at the time, another series that I knew none of houses for which I worked would even consider because one of the main characters was too old to fit the profile of what they believed sold.

Unknown to me, she sent those books to a new house, one which didn't have a profile or requirements. The house bought all four books. I loved working for Meteor and Kismet Publishing. The character that no one would have considered was very popular. Her name was Pippa and her author is Lacey Dancer.

When Meteor was sold to its biggest competitor, I decided for family reasons to retire from writing. I missed writing too much to stay retired. Computers, the internet and social media arrived and opened doors to new ideas and ways to publish.

I love a challenge and I really like breaking new ground. Is it easy? Absolutely not. There are more questions than answers some days.

For me, this new world of publishing is tailor made. I make my own rules, write my way, stories I like with characters that drive me nuts on a good day and make me crazy on a busy day. I love what I do. I especially love the freedom of doing what I do my way.

CONTACT THE AUTHOR

International, Award-Winning Romance and Suspense author, Sydney Clary a.k.a. Lacey Dancer, has written and published over 36 books over her lifetime that have been published in 20 different languages in over 100 countries. She is working on adding 20 or 30 more to the count as well as bringing her backlist into the 21st century. During her writing career she has garnered 2 Lifetime Achievement awards from the Romance Writers of America.

Email: laceydancerauthor@gmail.com
Website: https://laceydancer.com
Twitter: https://twitter.com/LaceyTheAuthor
Instagram: https://www.instagram.com/laceydancerauthor/
Facebook: https://www.facebook.com/BooksByLaceyDancer/
LinkedIn: https://www.linkedin.com/in/Lacey-Dancer-Author
YouTube: https://www.youtube.com/@laceydancerauthor
Pinterest: https://www.pinterest.com/laceydancerauthor/
Goodreads: https://www.goodreads.com/author/show/362798.Lacey_Dancer

OTHER BOOKS BY THIS AUTHOR

The Live Oak Series

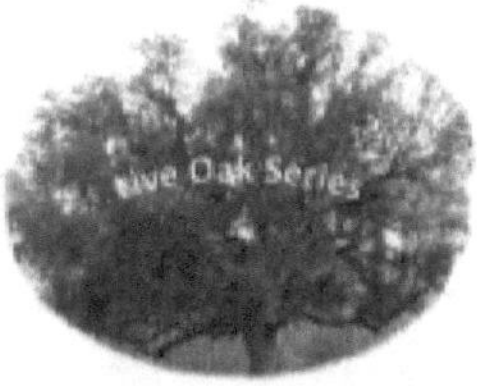

Live Oak is a real place. Small towns all over the country are struggling to keep their way of life and heritage intact and still survive in the 21st century. That is the background for the Live Oak Series, but the characters are the heart of the stories, their struggles, triumphs, and solutions to the twists and turns in life. Live Oak in my fictional world is filled with challenges and triumphs.

Every character in this series is fictional. Except two. Those two are Jennifer and Tina who appear in books three and four. These two friends of mine talked me into putting them in the story. We made a deal. Each had to create her own physical description. Each will have her own book. I am working on Jennifer's now.

A stalker sneaks into town to kill. Country justice comes in the form of an irate donkey named Jay.

A city woman who needs her lattes and shoe stores discovers the misadventures of tractors and barnyard animals that have no idea when to shut up in the morning. Normal people do not wake up at dawn.

The construction crew arrives to build a vision of the future for Live Oak. Mother Nature has other ideas with a hurricane on the east coast and a bomb on the west coast.

Add in a child escaping terrible abuse and neglect, a cranky judge, a sheriff who heads the local country band, and a wounded veteran who is not going to give up and the plot thickens with every book.

That doesn't count the three weddings to date and two more in the future.

Chase the Fire[1] - Book 1

Playing with Fire[2] - Book 2

Strike the Fire[3] - Book 3

Catch the Fire[4] - Book 4

Light the Fire[5] - Book 5

---

1. https://books2read.com/ChaseTheFireBook1
2. https://books2read.com/PlayingWithFireBook2
3. https://books2read.com/StrikeTheFireBook3
4. https://books2read.com/CatchTheFireBook4
5. https://books2read.com/Light-The-Fire-Book-5

The Pippa Series

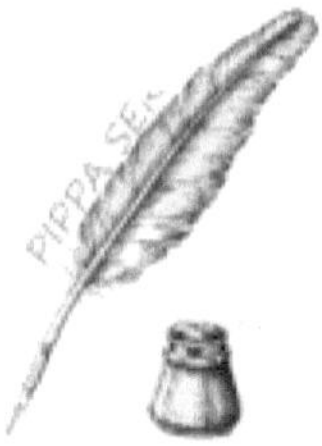

Pippa, an aunt, a friend, a writer. Following rules, unless they are her own, is so not on her agenda. She writes and values her solitude. Birthdays, specifically hers, are not to be celebrated. Have a permanent man in her life is a complication she can happily forgo. However, her relatives and friends might just need a little help in finding a life partner. And she loves a challenge.

Tragically injured, hiding from the world, her niece. Lorelei is the first to discover how ingenious a loving, determined woman can be. Pippa issues a challenge. The doctors are positive Lorelei will never walk again. Pippa dares Lorelei to prove them wrong. *"Come live with me and rebuild your life. Needing a place to recover, Lorelei accepts the challenge."*

When a workaholic male appears in the neighborhood, Pippa takes his measure and makes her plans. The impossible becomes very possible.

Pippa decides that her plans worked so well with Lorelei, she really must do something about her nephew, Jason. The Iceman faces the frozen wasteland of his life as Pippa adroitly maneuvers him into meeting Diana Diamond. Diana shuns the spotlight and Jason lives for it. Opposites are so much fun to match, especially as the sparks fly. Yes, she definitely has her hands full with these two but she is up for the challenge.

With two successes to her personal credit, Pippa decides on a trip, a thirteen-day cruise. Wow, Lilah is like a wounded creature, hiding from the media, shrinking from the least contact. Pippa reaches out even as she is discovering her own match in Joshua Luck.

Joshua is stunned at the woman who challenges and entices with every word, every move. Following her thought processes is like chasing a rabbit on steroids. Pippa is like no woman he has ever met. She makes her own rules, delves into lives, meddling, and arranging with such heart it is impossible not to admire her tactics even as he deals with his reaction to her.

She makes the rules, breaks the rules, and dares everyone with whom she comes in contact to reach for their every wish and dream. The bigger the challenge, the happier Pippa is. Impossible is a word she doesn't recognize, and no is a word she ignores.

What's a man to do with a woman like that? Marry her? Spend his life wondering what she will do next? Who will she decide needs her special matchmaking touch?

Choices[6] – Book 1

Diamonds and Ice[7] – Book 2

Thirteen Nights of Luck[8] – Book 3

6. https://books2read.com/ChoicesBook1
7. https://books2read.com/DiamondAndIceBook2
8. https://books2read.com/ThirteenNightsOfLuckBook3

The Truth Series

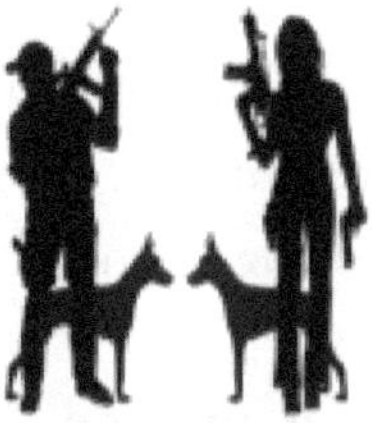

Felicity Ramsey could be anyone. Your best friend? Your worst enemy? She moved through the shadows without making a sound, no warning given. She was a hunter. She had been taught from the cradle how to seek her prey and make the kill. She hated killing but she killed. Her prey was the monster who could escape the law, could hide in plain sight from justice.

Evidence and alibis could be manufactured. Governmental lines could become borders over which the law could not pass. The monsters were many. She was just one. But there were more. The human weapons trained and formed by governments to fight wars with no real winners. Men and women who could not forget the lethal skills they had learned and reenter the world that they had fought to protect.

Skye Farm and Skye/Sea were born, created on her own private mountain. The Farm was home and haven to those lost warriors who no longer had a place in civilization. Their skills and training were sought and valued by the government and the private sector.

Secure on her mountain, Felicity sought the monsters the law could not catch or exact retribution. She worked alone until one man; Ace Faulkner faced her in a room with a friend beaten to near death lying on the floor between them.

Ace had a choice. Shoot to kill? Or holster his gun?

Felicity had a choice. Trust the man? Or save the woman at her feet?

One choice made. Two guns laid aside to save a life.

Two loners, working together.

An expected phone call on a line that no one should have, creates a threat to everything that Felicity has built, the Farm, the Ranch and all those who work and live on her three mountains. A code 'blue' thrown over all of Skye/Sea. An infiltration by foreign interests in Washington, an accidental death of a loved one of one of their own has created more questions rather than answers.

In the air, on the sea and on the land, the teams gear up to protect their home and find the traitors in their government who profited from their acts of treason.

Truth Kills[9] – Book 1

Truth Tells[10] – Book 2

Truth Wins[11] – Book 3

---

9. https://books2read.com/TruthKillsBook1

10. https://books2read.com/TruthTellsBook2

11. https://books2read.com/TruthWinsBook3

BOOK BY SYDNEY CLARY

Are you facing the task of care for an aging relative, a child or loved one through a serious illness? This book is a real-life approach to handling the multitude of problems that crop up each day.

In your home, in a care facility and all the variations of caregiving locations, there are ways to help those who matter to you and help yourself survive the stress and strain of caregiving.

- How to wait in waiting rooms.
- How to find a new location for your loved one when the present situation no longer meets the needs of your relative or friend.
- How to handle medical insurance.
- How to handle home care.
- How to resolve problems with medical staff.
- How to get bills paid.

There are answers to these issues and many others, real-life answers that work. Need an idea or new avenue for that dead-end you are facing as a caregiver.

The goal of this book is to provide those answers, those suggestions. Examples of use are in every chapter, real people dealing with problems and solutions. Some will make you smile; some will make you cry but each will show what can be done as you face this demanding and rewarding task in your own life.

Caregiving: Real Life Answers[1]

1. https://books2read.com/CareGivingByClary

BACK BOOK LISTING FOR LACEY DANCER

Only available at used paperback book outlets*(enhanced and revised)

Single novel

Sunlight on Shadows (1991)

Baby Makes Five (1992)

Starke-McGuire

Silent Enchantment (1990) – Re-released and enhanced titled – Choices*

Diamond On Ice (1991) – Re-released and enhanced titled – Diamond and Ice*

13 Days of Luck (1991)

Flight of the Swan (1992)

Forever Joy (1993)

Lightning Strikes Twice (1993)

His Woman's Gift (1993)

Many Faces of Love (2003)

St. James Series

Silke (1996)

Caprice (1996)

Leora (1996)

Noelle (1996)

Check out her Wiki Page: https://en.wikipedia.org/wiki/Lacey_Dancer

www.ingramcontent.com/pod-product-compliance
Lightning Source LLC
LaVergne TN
LVHW100317210926
848480LV00003B/1155